- 'Brilliant, readable, witty and wise, this book offers the first systematic Darwinian explanation for cancer. Only rarely do comprehensive knowledge, vivid historical anecdotes, the latest scientific findings, and original ideas come together with such literary flourish'

  R Nesse (University of Michigan. Author of '*Why We Get Sick*')

- 'This is the first book on cancer that unites insights from the entire spectrum of biology. It's also fun to read. As a tour guide, Greaves is clever but not snooty, deep but still accessible'

  P W Ewald and G M Cochran in *American Scientist*

- 'The book is as much a cultural chronicle as a biology lesson, and Greaves marshalls literature, history and his own puckish if macabre sense of humor to tell this complex story'

  J Newman in *New York Times Book Review*

- 'This is one of the most readable books I have ever opened and was as good as a thriller! Anyone with an interest in cancer should read this book'

  H Mercer in *Nursing Standard*

- 'A personal, high-spirited narrative by an experienced and knowledgeable cancer researcher. By clearing away the intellectual camouflage guarding evolution and cancer, Greaves makes the topic accessible to both general readers and specialists'

  D Shibata in *New England Journal of Medicine*

- 'An absolute delight'

  S Ohno (Beckman Institute, California. Author of '*Evolution by Gene Duplication*')

- 'Few exponents of the field (*Darwinian medicine*) have used the insights of evolution so powerfully. Cancer. The Evolutionary Legacy is at once a work of high-level popularization and an original contribution to the scientific literature on cancer'

  W F Bynum in *Times Literary Supplement*

- '. . . (a) view of the cancer problem that is unmatched in scope and depth by any other popular science book currently available – explanations that are models of clarity. Highly recommended to specialist and non-specialist readers alike'

  H R Baillie-Johnson in *Clinical Oncology*

- '. . . the book is a great success; throughout the text, he shows time and time again how an evolutionary angle can provide stimulation and fresh food for thought'

  J L Lee in *Bulletin of the Royal College of Pathologists*

- 'This is the perfect book for the dedicated oncologist – or even interested laymen – to take on holiday'
  J Wellbreak in *Cancer Topics*

- 'A meticulous scientific explanation of cancer in all its wretched manifestations, cast in the light of evolutionary biology'
  in *Kirkus Reviews*

- 'refreshing . . ., well researched and lucidly proposed arguments. A stimulating read'
  M Okasha in *Lancet Oncology*

- 'An extremely attractive, thought provoking yet easy to read text in which Darwinian medicine is applied to human cancer'
  F Alexander in *Journal of Perinatal and Paediatric Epidemiology*

- '. . . written in a witty and easy to read style – the book provides a fascinating and enlightening insight into the evolution of cancer, its causes and treatment'
  G Johnson in *Family Practice Journal*

- 'I would highly recommend this book. Mel Greaves provides anyone interested in cancer with a real treat of facts, speculation and rare anecdotes, to explore the origin of cancer'
  C Boshoff in *British Journal of Cancer*

- 'a cleverly paced and extremely informative guide to current thinking about evolutionary biology and cancer . . . worth a rackful of popular paperbacks'
  D Park in *The Lancet*

- 'Conveyed with wit, fluency and authenticity . . . beautifully put into historical context, it (*cancer*) can rarely have been described with such aplomb'
  N J Maitland in *Heredity*

- 'This important book is well worth the read'
  L Nunney in *Quarterly Review of Biology*

- 'The word 'entertaining' might seem out of place in the context of cancer, but Greaves manages to be just that without insensitivity . . . (he) has performed a huge service in writing a book that is both accurate and accessible. It should be piled high in supermarkets and distributed, at taxpayers' expense, with packs of cigarettes'
  C M Steel in *Nature Medicine*

- 'The time is ripe for a book that embraces the science and the art (*of cancer causes, treatment and research*) in a non-patronising style, and with Cancer. The Evolutionary Legacy, Mel Greaves has succeeded brilliantly . . . (a) magnificent book'
  R C F Leonard in *Journal of the Royal Society of Medicine*

CANCER

The evolutionary legacy

MEL GREAVES

Professor of Cell Biology,
at the Institute of Cancer Research, London

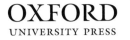

OXFORD
UNIVERSITY PRESS

OXFORD

UNIVERSITY PRESS

Great Clarendon Street, Oxford OX2 6DP

Oxford University Press is a department of the University of Oxford. It
furthers the University's objective of excellence in research, scholarship,
and education by publishing worldwide in

Oxford New York

Athens Auckland Bangkok Bogotá Buenos Aires Calcutta Cape Town
Chennai Dar es Salaam Delhi Florence Hong Kong Istanbul Karachi
Kuala Lumpur Madrid Melbourne Mexico City Mumbai Nairobi Paris
São Paulo Singapore Taipei Tokyo Toronto Warsaw

with associated companies in Berlin Ibadan

Oxford is a registered trade mark of Oxford University Press in the UK and
in certain other countries

Published in the United States by Oxford University Press Inc., New York

British Library Cataloguing in Publication Data
Data available

Library of Congress Cataloging in Publication Data

ISBN 0 19 262834 8 (pbk)
1 3 5 7 9 10 8 6 4 2

Typeset in Minion by Footnote Graphics, Warminster, Wilts
Printed in Great Britain on acid-free paper
by T. J. International Ltd, Padstow

PREFACE

Science provides us with one way of viewing the world we live in. For its practitioners, curiosity is a propellant but it helps to be both optimistic and a tad naïve if you are trying to distil a clear picture from natural world phenomena in which the dimensions of space and time are beyond our experience and where the richness of the tapestry can so easily obscure vision. Getting to grips with such complexities is what it's all about and for some of us, this challenge is most inviting when it touches on the human condition.

Cancer is one such puzzle, tantalizingly inviting a solution but ever elusive, belligerent, and indecipherable. Or is it? There is now a plausible and coherent explanation for this capricious disease that makes sense and this book is an attempt to describe it. It's a narrative of history, of geography, of molecular shenanigans, of human foibles, and lotteries. But most of all, it's about evolution.

It is my personal view that the perspective that best explains the puzzle of cancer is an evolutionary or Darwinian one. Only a few years ago this would, I suspect, have fallen on stony ground. But fortunately the way has been cleared. I can't turn on my radio or television without hearing vociferous arguments about genes and evolution, usually coupled with cloning, sex, or religion. Evolution, and neo-Darwinian biology, we are reliably informed by the pundits, can illuminate everything from the oddities of our body parts to our language capacity, psychological traits, and even our economies – and especially, perhaps, our illnesses.

Randolph Nesse and George Williams coined the term 'Darwinian medicine' for this new perspective on why we get sick. Darwin is certainly enjoying something of a rapturous encore, preceded on stage by the wizardry of Watson and Crick, and then much heralded by George Williams, Richard Dawkins, Steve Jones, Daniel Dennett, and other eloquent and enthusiastic comperes.

It is the power of molecular genetics that has fuelled this new biological view of humanity. But the vision is poverty-stricken if the picture in the puzzle is a one-dimensional look at genes. Our biology is much more multilayered and interesting than this. Still, genes sit at the centre of this cancer story as part of an extraordinary web of interactions in a great game of chance, with players and rules bequeathed by evolution. Cancer is ubiquitous in nature and in a sense a natural part of nature. But there is something special about our human predicament and the high incidence of cancer in our societies. It has to do with how we have changed the rules of evolutionary games. How we've become entrapped in a nature–nurture mismatch.

What I hope this Darwinian perspective provides is a plausible framework for tackling the big questions in cancer that concern us all. Why does it exist at all? Why doesn't a healthy body deal with it? Why is it so common? Why are there so many risk factors? Why do the best therapeutic efforts usually fail? What exactly is it? What can we do about it? And – why me? Some old illusions of simplicity, on cause and cure in particular, have had to be dumped and some of the answers, as astute observers of the scientific scene would have anticipated, are counter-intuitive at first glance but make striking sense once comprehended in their proper context.

Cancer is one of the major afflictions of developed societies. The fact that causation is multifactorial and involves both very ancient and more recent evolutionary legacies implies that there are no easy answers. But we will have new options to consider in terms of early diagnosis, biological therapy, and especially prevention. The potential implications for the future are very considerable – for genetic screening and counselling, risk assessment, novel therapeutic strategies, the commercial biotechnology enterprise, health service organization and costs, and, perhaps most significantly of all, our social behaviour.

What's on offer here is still just one 'way of seeing' – out of many perspectives that could be preferred. My agenda is straightforward and I trust transparent: I want to explore the extent to which an evolutionary and historical look over our shoulder can inform the key issues we face in cancer. I have no expectations that it will provide a complete or exclusive interpretation or offer solace to patients, but I'm optimistic that it can help us to see the problem in a clearer light.

Scientific and medical publications can be irredeemably technical, dry, and impenetrable with narrative style, speculation, anecdote, and humour strictly verboten and metaphors rationed. One of the reasons I've written this book is that it has provided me with a vehicle to escape these professional strictures. So it is somewhat self-indulgent, but hopefully not at the expense of general interest, accuracy, and reasoned judgement. It should be clear what is accepted wisdom and what is speculation. Certainly there is a lot of uncertainty in it and plenty that appears paradoxical. I've simplified some very complex or technical issues and tried to avoid an excess of caveats and qualifications that more prudent scientists might append to cover themselves. I've also kept named accreditation, references, and notes to a minimum. There's an obvious risk here of irritating fellow scientists and expert reviewers. My apologies for this, but the book has not been written for the professionals.

MG
London, 1999

ACKNOWLEDGEMENTS

Many people have helped me in the writing of this book by reading sections of it and offering criticisms and suggestions. I am grateful in particular to Freda Alexander, David Dearnaley, Richard Doll, Tariq Enver, Tom Greaves, Barry Gusterson, Andrew Lister, Chris Marshall, and Robin Weiss. Nick Day, Maria Elena Cabrera, Sonia Guillen, Faith Ho, Richard Houlston, Richard Montali, David Onions, Shizu Saki, Mike Stratton, and David Wood kindly provided me with helpful information. Chris Priest helped with artwork and several colleagues provided illustrations; they are acknowledged under photographic credits. Miss Gay Davies and the Library staff at the Institute of Cancer Research were particularly helpful in accessing both current and historical sources of information on cancer.

For the past 25 years, I have been the beneficiary of support from charitable cancer research organizations that have allowed me the luxury of doing what I find most interesting and the rewards of joining in expeditions into the jungle that is cancer. Many thanks therefore to the Institute of Cancer Research, The Leukaemia Research Fund, and the Imperial Cancer Research Fund.

Susan Harrison and her colleagues at Oxford University Press were very supportive throughout. I thank Barbara Deverson for her excellent secretarial help. Any errors, as the saying goes, are all mine.

For Jo

CONTENTS

FIGURE ACKNOWLEDGEMENTS

Figure 2.1 Portrait of Ferrante I of Arragon in *Adorazione dei Magi* by M. Cardisco. Kindly provided by Drs A. Marchetti and G. Fornaciari.

Figure 8.2 Kindly provided by Professor M A Konerding.

Figure 8.3 Kindly provided by Professor R Ott.

Figure 10.1 From author's laboratory. Previously published in Price CM *et al. Blood*, 1992, **80**: 1035 and in *Institute of Cancer Research/Royal Marsden Hospital Annual Scientific Report 1991/92*.

Figure 10.2 By kind permission of J Workman.

Figure 11.2 Picture of Napoleon is from portrait entitled *St Helena. The Last Phase* by James Sant. Courtesy of the Glasgow Museums: Art Gallery and Museum, Kelvingrove.

Figure 13.1 By kind permission of J Chase.

Figure 14.1 From *A History of Smoking* by Count Corti, 1931.

Figure 14.2 From Reddy DG *et al. Cancer*, 1960, **13**: 263. With permission.

Figure 15.1 (Also Plate 2 and back cover image) From Leiden University. MS Vossios lat3, fol 90v.

Figure 15.2 From *A History of Pathology* by ER Long, Dover Publications, 1965.

Figure 19.1 From Urteaga O and Pack GT. *Cancer*, 1966, **19**: 609. With permission.

Figure 21.1 Left and centre pictures from *Dangerous Trades* by T Oliver (1902) J Murray Press, London (pictures derived originally from studies of HT Butlin, 1880).

Right picture from London Tower Hamlets Local History Library archive.

Figure 23.1 Image of roulette wheel courtesy of Cary Designs.

Figure 25.1 By kind permission of S Harris.

PART ONE

CANCER: ANCIENT LEGACIES AND MODERN MYTHS

No man, even under torture,
Can say exactly what a tumor is.

J Ewing, 1916

CHAPTER 1

PERPLEXED? YOU SHOULD BE

Allow me to start with the bad news will you? Statistics. Around one in three of us will at some time have an unwelcomed diagnosis of cancer, providing common ground between presidents, movie stars, bishops, athletes, Nobel prize winners, Jew and gentile, black and white, wealthy and destitute. Every day, around 1500 Americans die of the disease and, needless to say, vastly more non-Americans. Worldwide, over eight million new cancer diagnoses are delivered each year. It's geographically and ethnically ubiquitous, and it's a big problem. Something of an acute problem in Western societies relishing wealth, health, and longevity, anticipating the quick fix and perplexed by the lack of it. In the developed world, with the eradication of infection and malnutrition as major causes of mortality, cancer has, largely by default, become more prominent as a life-threatening illness in children, although its frequency in the young remains very low.

The illness we call cancer has extraordinarily diverse features including its causation, underlying pathology, clinical symptoms, therapeutic response, and outcome or chance of cure. In a sense, every patient's cancer is unique, which is part of the difficulty. In so far as it is *a* disease, it is a collection of very many (a thousand or so) disorders of cell and tissue function that have one special biological property in common – *the territorial expansion of a mutant clone*.

Cancer can be a thoroughly horrible illness. Capricious and insidious it may be but our perception of the problem is in no small measure distorted by the label itself – 'cancer' (a gift from the Greeks). The name is, for a medical condition, uniquely evocative and has helped engender a pervasive and frightening notion of what it means to have the illness. It's a shame we cannot deinvent the word. As Susan Sontag vividly described in her book *Illness As Metaphor*, cancer has become enshrined in its own mythology as an obscene and demonic predator, an invincible grim reaper. It is no surprise that a diagnosis of cancer can so easily promote exaggerated fear. A fear of inevitable outcome. A fear exacerbated either by guilt that one's own habits, some life-enhancing and pleasurable, may be to blame or by anger that some filthy and unregulated industrial enterprise is the villain. And, as if that wasn't bad enough, cancer may hijack parts of our anatomy that we would rather not talk about, at least when they are not in perfect working order. Pain, shame, and a dash of anger make a rotten cocktail.

This state of alarm is, in many respects, understandable but it is un-questionably fuelled by ignorance, ill-conceived claims, and inconsistent but striking anecdotes, and is reinforced by what is perceived to be a startling lack of progress in control or eradication. Breakthroughs are forever 'just around the corner' and an increasingly more sceptical public is tempted to turn to alternative medicine. The national cost of treatment, research, and lost income, as well as the physical and emotional burden to patients and their families is enormous.

The reality is that treatment for cancer can be nasty and toxic, and doctors and scientists have overall done a rather poor job in explaining why this is so and what the underlying problems are. And yet, there have been real im-provements in clinical management, a revolution in our understanding of the underlying biology of cancer, and a much more sophisticated appreciation of the multiple factors involved in causation. At last we have some understanding of what it really is, why the complexity exists. This new knowledge explains past failures and, in the longer term, offers a plausible route to control through earlier detection and intervention, more efficacious, less toxic treatment, and, last but not least, prevention. The demon is ripe for exorcism.

We now know from advances in molecular genetics of the past 25 years that cancer develops as a chromosomal gene disorder in single cells. But it is different and more complex than the 5000 or so other human genetic diseases that arise as inherited, single-gene traits. It is also different from the disease paradigm the public most readily understands, or rather misunderstands, of common infectious illnesses, caused by individual culprit micro-organisms and that are, on the whole, amenable to treatment or prevention. The simple formula, infection with X = disease Y: treat with Z is an illusion that disguises a more complex aetiology. Susan Sontag in castigating the mystification of cancer also indulges in inappropriate or superficial analogies (with tuberculosis) and wishful thinking – in supposing that the escape from this dilemma must lie in simple, singular, and exclusive explanations of cause and cure. But she is not alone in anticipating a straightforward relationship between cause and effect.[1] The notion is pervasive, especially in Western societies. What has engendered it? Potential explanations include the philosophical determinism of Descartes, Leibniz, and Newtonian physics, and, at a more influential level perhaps, Hollywood movies. These provide the rationale and precedents for one-dimensional thinking: linear, all or none relationships between causes and effects, villains and victims and seduction by simple explanations and solutions, however illusory.

But cancer and indeed most other diseases are inherently more complex. And this complexity is not just an oddity of our ailments, it's an essential feature of the biological worlds that our genes, cells, and bodies inhabit – of the way living things work. This inevitable but frequently ignored difficulty has frustrated both sustained attempts at eradication and efforts to explain the nature of cancer without resorting to superficiality. Simple explanations won't wash. Worse still, erroneous perceptions of the existence of *a* cause and the possibility of *a* cure have fuelled unrealistic expectations. There is no singular cause. Ionizing radiation is the only known cause of breast cancer and was similarly indicted for leukaemia. But it clearly isn't *the* cause of these cancers or even involved in anything but a small minority of them. Of course it's confusing. But we have a need to pin the blame on somebody, to nail something. Nobody knows and everyone knows. It's bad bile. It's bad habits. It's bad bosses. It's bad genes. It's bad luck. It certainly is bad luck. It's the air we breathe, the water we drink, the food we eat. All of these and none of these.

The painful reality is that there is no holy grail, no magic cure-all bullet, and no quick fix. And the paradox is that all the complexity, now that the fog is lifting, has a coherent pattern and makes a great deal of sense. And, as often when seen in retrospect, it is difficult to imagine how it could have been otherwise. Demystifying the disease is to travel over a new and more realistic landscape. It's not the easiest of journeys but it's the only ticket worth having.

CHAPTER 2

THE KING OF NAPLES AND OTHER SILENT WITNESSES

In some respects, cancer sits alongside heart attacks, strokes, obesity, neurodegenerative disease of older age, and AIDS as a very twentieth-century disease, an integral part of our culture. As were, in our not too distant past, bubonic plague, syphilis, and tuberculosis. But is it a new affliction? Call the King of Naples.

Ferrante I of Arragon and King of Naples (see Fig. 2.1) died obese, aged 63, in 1494. His body was mummified by embalming and, in common with several compatriots of noble descent, was placed in a wooden sarcophagus in the Abbey of San Domenico Maggiore in Naples. Necropsy of the exhumed body revealed what appeared to be a relatively well-preserved tumour in the pelvic region. Italian scientists from the Institute of Pathology, Pisa University, made sections of the tumour, scrutinized the pathology, and surmised that it was probably a type of cancer called adenocarcinoma, possibly derived from the large intestine. They then performed a sensitive molecular test for a gene mutation commonly found today in this type of cancer. The test, called the polymerase chain reaction, can detect as little as a single copy of a gene (or fragment of a gene) using an amplification method that has become the mainstay of molecular pathology and forensic science laboratories. The human gene involved is called *RAS* and the cancer tissue from Ferrante I did indeed have the precise mutation in *RAS* anticipated from present-day cancers. A diagnostic *tour de force*, albeit a little late for the patient.

Still older human remains provide evidence for the antiquity of cancer, though degradation of DNA has removed the molecular fingerprint from the scene of the crime. The presence of putative bone tumours (osteosarcomas or bone-seeking cancers spreading from other tissues) has been inferred from malformations and lesions of skeletal remains from neolithic times, as well as in pre-Columbian native Americans, and in medieval Europe. The most dramatic of these, discovered in Stanlake in Oxfordshire[3], is an enormous bony growth and probable osteosarcoma belonging to a young Saxon male.

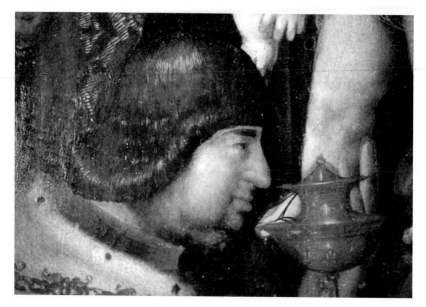

Figure 2.1 Ferrante I of Arragon and King of Naples.[2]

Whilst alternative diagnoses, post-mortem degeneration, or ossification following injury or infection are possible, many, perhaps around a hundred in total, skulls and long bones (femurs) examined have structures compatible with primary bone tumours or lesions highly suggestive of cancer that has spread or metastasized from other sites. The most common forms are described as benign ivory osteomas of the skull. Seventeen such cases derived from skulls of British origin from neolithic to Saxon times have been described. A similar survey of remains from Pecos Pueblo Indians revealed 13 such cases in a total of 581 skulls examined.

Malignant cancers are more difficult to identify in skeletal remains but the skull lesions of several specimens are highly suggestive of bone-seeking cancers such as those of breast, multiple myeloma, or melanoma which produce characteristic bone damage. The oldest of such specimens include a female skull from the Bronze Age (1900–1600 BC) which the author of the report speculated originated from a breast tumour, and a possible case of multiple myeloma in a skull from the fourth century in Kentucky. Other remarkable examples include mummified skeletal remains from Incas in Peru that may be as ancient as 2400 years old and which house multiple lesions characteristic of disseminated malignant melanoma. This may seem odd given that the incumbent indigenous people of the same region have very low rates of melanoma, a cancer more generally associated with excess UV light exposure and skin burning in pale-skinned Caucasians. On the other hand, as we'll see later, it may be telling us something very interesting about the migrant groups that colonized the Americas.

The oldest possible malignant tumour in a hominid is in a fossil jaw bone (the Kanam mandible) discovered in Kenya in 1932 by Louis Leakey. The unwitting donor of the archaeological treasure was either an *Australopithecus* or a *Homo erectus*. George Stathopolous, a Greek oncologist, suggested that the tumour might have been a Burkitt's lymphoma, a type of cancer endemic in current East Africa and that commonly develops in the jaw. It is unlikely that this can be proven one way or the other but it's a tantalizing thought that this disease might have existed some one to two million years before the British surgeon, Dr Denis Burkitt, uncovered it for Western eyes and gave it a label.

Egyptian papyri written between 1500 BC and 3000 BC refer to tumours of the breast. The Ebers papyrus contains a description of loathsome large tumours of the leg. The tumours were said to '... call with a loud voice to thee "it is a tumour of the god Xensu. Do thou nothing against thee."' Michael Shimkin who provided an excellent illustrated review of this early history of cancers suggested that although the god Xensu tumour might not be a tumour at all, the description given would fit Kaposi's sarcoma, a form of cancer currently endemic in Egypt, the Eastern Mediterranean in general, and parts of Africa, and also common in patients with AIDS. A few cases of bone tumours and possible nasopharyngeal cancers in mummified Egyptian bodies from up to 5000 years ago have also been described.

Two particularly intriguing cases of probable cancer in ancient Egyptian skeletons reside in the Turin Anthropology Institute. These were both males, one aged 20–25 years, the other around 60 years. Both have very unusual skeletal malformations including split ribs and abnormal digits which are characteristic of Gorlin's syndrome. This was first described as a distinct entity in 1960 (by Gorlin and Golz) and its striking feature, other than multiple bone and tissue irregularities, is the high prevalence of several types of benign and malignant tumours including multiple skin cancers, providing the disorder with its descriptive name, nevoid basal cell carcinoma. Predisposition to Gorlin's syndrome is inherited via a gene which has recently been molecularly cloned and identified as the human evolutionary counterpart of a gene in *Drosophila* fruit flies called *patched*. Now it so happens that the same gene, *Patched*, is very commonly present as a mutant gene in the single most common form of cancer, a non-melanoma skin cancer called basal cell carcinoma. Here, the gene is not inherited in a mutant form but undergoes mutation in a single skin cell, probably as a consequence of exposure to UV light. Given the rarity of the Gorlin syndrome gene in contemporary Western societies (less than 1 in 50 000) it seems very likely that the two Egyptian skeletons are related individuals, perhaps father and son.

The ancient Greeks are credited with being the first to recognize cancer as a distinct disease and coined the terms carcinos and carcinoma (both meaning crab), the Latinized version of which we use today. This description was however applied both to ulcerating tumours and to non-cancerous conditions including inflammatory reactions, cysts, and haemorrhoids. Hippocrates (460–370 BC) described cancers of the breast, nasopharynx, stomach, skin, cervix, and rectum.[4] Hydatidiform mole was also recognized in ancient Greece and Rome. This is a biologically unique tumour of the uterus that we will hear more about later.

Accessible cancers, such as those of the breast, were removed surgically, the resultant wounds and unextirpated superficial tumours being treated by the application of coal tar pastes or herbal poisons including hemlock, belladonna, and arsenic – a harbinger of what was to come two thousand years later. For less accessible cancers, Hippocrates had wise advice to offer. His Aphorism number 38 reads: '... it is better not to apply any treatment in cases of occult cancer; for, if treated, the patients die quickly, but if not treated they hold out for a long time.'[4]

Galen, a Greek physician practising in Rome in the second century, is regarded by many as the founding father of clinical medicine and the first oncologist. He described in some detail the appearance of cancers of many different organs including the female reproductive tract and the intestines, but especially in the breast which he recorded as the commonest cancer. In this context, he also offers us a plausible derivation of the label 'cancer': '... and on the breasts we often saw tumours resembling exactly the animal cancer (crab). And just as the animal's legs are on either side of the body, so do the veins stretched by the unnatural tumour resemble cancer in shape.' Galen followed Hippocrates in believing that superficial tumours, such as those of the breast, could be cured by surgical removal, whereas abortive attempts at removal of internal or deep-seated cancer caused only misery and accelerated demise of the patients. Interestingly, in the context of our current understanding of cancer, he emphasized that breast cancers were only curable by surgery before they grew beyond a certain size. Whether mastectomy as practised in ancient Greece, in Rome, and throughout subsequent European history really was curative we cannot know but the ninth-century Arab surgeon Abdul Qasim provides us with an honest and salutary quote: 'I for one never could cure one single case, nor do I know anybody else who succeeded in doing so.'

Ayurvedic medical books from India from 2000–2500 years ago describe the identification and treatment of tumours (Arbuda). Metastatic or disseminated cancers were also recognized. Tumours of the oral cavity, pharynx, and oesophagus were particularly common, as in present-day South East Asia. Oral cavity cancers, including those of the tongue, buccal cavity, and palate may have been associated with the chewing of betal quid, as in current day India. Internal cancers such as those of the colon, liver, and stomach were not recorded, which is perhaps not surprising, but the apparent lack of breast cancer is striking when compared to the contemporaneous description of these as relatively common female cancers in Greece.

Chinese folklore suggests that the oesophageal or throat cancer has an extraordinarily long history throughout the Eastern world. It was recorded as common in Persia by the eleventh century and was probably so much earlier. Currently, in certain regions of northern China, up to 10 per cent of adult men and women develop oesophageal cancer. The explanation as we shall see later is predominantly dietary, but what is remarkable is that the disease has, according to local folklore, been prevalent in the same areas for more than 2000 years.

Hippocrates, and later Galen, both ascribed cancer to an excess of black bile. This was in accord with the humoral theories of disease that predominated in ancient Greece and Rome and seemingly endorsed in the bloody appearance of many tumours caused by vascularization and ulceration. Fertile ground for metaphors? The encapsulation of cancer via grim metaphors dates back to ancient Greece and Rome, as does the reciprocal literary gambit of describing pervasive, insidious, corrupting, or evil activities as cancerous. In his poem *Metamorphoses*, the Latin poet Ovid refers to the rampant jealousy of an Athenian girl for her sister as just like cancer – 'an irremediable ailment taking over and corrupting the body'. In the same vein, but in the Bible, we have St Paul's disapproval of godless people as those 'whose words will eat as does the canker'.

Cancer then is an illness as old as *Homo sapiens* and indeed, very much older. The Kanam mandible isn't in fact the record holder for the oldest identified tumour. That prize currently rests with a haemangioma (a benign tumour of blood vessels) and another cancer of uncertain type whose unique imprints were identified in dinosaur bones from the Jurassic period, more than 150 million years ago. One wouldn't expect to find fossilized remains of more malignant cancers but when we come to consider the essential biological nature of cancer, you'll see that it reflects such an intrinsic feature of multicellular creatures that we can be reasonably confident that benign and malignant growths have been around for half a billion years or so. It's just that no pathologists have been around to label them as such. All five vertebrate classes of animal, plus molluscs and some other invertebrates living today, develop some forms of cancer, albeit at modest frequencies and sometimes suspiciously linked to human activities. We humans invented the label cancer but not the condition.

CHAPTER 3

SOOT, CIVILIZATION, AND NEUROSES

> May we, then, infer that, as has more than once been contended, cancer, like insanity, follows in the wake of civilization.
>
> *(Walter Hayle Walshe, Professor of Pathological Anatomy, University College, London, 1846)*

What then of the commonly held view that cancer is a product of industrialized societies? The idea has a strong philosophical connection with the oft repeated lament, associated with Jean Jacques Rousseau in particular, that with 'civilization' humans have lost touch with nature and are paying a price in terms of common diseases. More specifically, with cancer, the argument derives from epidemiological observations on links between industrial occupations and cancer (that of cancer of the scrotum in chimney sweeps by Percival Pott in 1775 being the best-known historical precedent). Around a hundred years ago, the hazards of skin cancer following occupational exposure to tars, oils, and x-rays were identified – all very much a product of technical, industrial, and commercial advances.

But even before these cancerous activities were prevalent, cancer was widely regarded as a modern disease. Nineteenth-century European doctors noted that cancer was uncommon in 'the savage races', by which they mostly referred to black Africans. Dr Livingstone in his missionary travels in Africa noted that the natives were troubled with fatty and fibrous tumours, but cancer itself was unknown. Similarly, nineteenth-century surgeons and physicians in Europe and the USA were impressed by the apparent rarity of cancers, and especially breast cancer, in Indians (in Calcutta for example), North Africans (in Algeria), and native Americans.

The distinguished Professor Walter Walshe was convinced that a stressful modern lifestyle was to blame for cancer. And in this respect the learned professor had interesting prophylactic advice to offer parents with respect to the choice of profession for their offspring. Law, medicine, and diplomacy were to be avoided, as should the speculation-ridden life of a merchant, banker, or stockbroker. The best chance of escaping cancer, Walshe preferred, was for men to join the armed forces or the church and for women to become governesses.

Prominent surgeons and physicians of the eighteenth and nineteenth century in Europe regarded cancer not only as a 'modern' stress-related disease but as predominantly an illness of women. Some of them also thought they knew why this was the case:

> Women are more subject to cancerous disorders than Men, especially such Women that are of sedentary, melancholic Disposition of Mind, and meet with such Disasters in Life, as occasion much trouble and Grief.

(Richard Guy, 1759)

These and other speculations on cancer causation by surgeons of the seventeenth to nineteenth centuries were, to some extent, a legacy of Galen's much earlier advocacy of constitutional melancholy as the underlying problem. The idea that personality might somehow be directly linked to cancer causation persisted into the twentieth century and the age of psychoanalysis. There is, therefore, a touch of irony in the suggestion that suppressed emotions were responsible for Sigmund Freud's cancer. Freud consumed around twenty cigars a day for most of his adult life. It might not be just coincidental therefore that he developed a lethal cancer in his mouth and jaw. Fellow psychoanalyst, Wilhem Reich, had another explanation however. His 'cancer research', inspired, so he tells, by Freud's illness, led to his Cancer Biopathy Theory (1948). From this comes the simple and obvious explanation that Freud's cancer was the consequence of emotional or psychic resignation and his constant biting down with his jaw as a substitute outlet for his repressed emotions. Well, in a way may be it was, but this is a serious misreading of the causal pathway. And it still has its adherents today. Yes, it's your personality that's to blame. It sounds like a Woody Allen aphorism and few take it seriously. Such psychobabble however was particularly popular in medical circles throughout the nineteenth century. The distinguished English surgeon, Herbert Snow, had much to say on this score, encapsulated with some eloquence in his 1891 publications *The Proclivity of Women to Cancerous Diseases* and *Cancer in its Relations to Insanity*. I'm saving some of his more deliciously politically incorrect sentiments until we come to consider the possible causes of breast cancer later in this book.

But irrespective of possible causal mechanisms, what do we know of the incidence levels of cancers prior to the twentieth century in Europe? The relative prevalence of breast and uterine or cervical cancer has been reiterated in many historical medical records since the Galen era, but few provide any insight into actual incidence. One of the outstanding surgeons of the eighteenth century, John Hunter, was very familiar with cancer. Much of his experience is distilled into his published lectures on the principles of surgery in which he states that cancer most commonly attacks the conglomerate glands, and first the breast[5]. Hunter does not mention cancer of the lung or colon, so we might assume that they were less common than breast cancer or other cancers that he refers to (those of the uterus, as well as lips, nose, testicles, and, somewhat surprisingly, pancreas).

The Dutch surgeon, Adrian Helvetius, practising in Paris at the end of the seventeenth century, performed both lumpectomy and mastectomy for breast cancer, which he claimed were curative. He also boasted that his father, a surgeon in The Hague, had operated on more than two thousand breast cancers. The eminent French surgeon, Alfred Valpeau, similarly claimed to have personally seen over one thousand cases of breast cancer in his practice during the first part of the nineteenth century. It was during this period that the first hospitals dedicated to cancer were built, in Rheims in 1740 (sponsored by the Canon of the cathedral) and later in London, in 1828, the Royal Free and Cancer (now Royal Marsden) Hospital.

Some idea of the relative frequency of breast and other cancers 200 years ago comes from the first statistical analysis of deaths from cancer – in men and women in Verona between 1760 and 1839 by Rigoni-Stern. Strikingly, there were 994 female deaths compared with only 142 males and of the female cases, approximately one third were breast and one third uterine cancer. We do not know whether there was any strong bias in recording these mortality data, nevertheless, the predominance of female cancers is remarkable. Rigoni-Stern also estimated cancer rates per 10 000 population at different ages and relative cancer incidence by comparing cancer deaths to total deaths. The total male plus female cancer death count for the period he surveyed was 1136 – only 0.75 per cent of the total 150 673 deaths. Accepting that cancer will have been underdiagnosed and most individuals would have died at a relatively young age, this still suggests a low rate compared with more recent times. Rigoni-Stern made another very pertinent observation that we will hear more of later: that whereas nuns were much more likely to die of breast cancer than married women, the opposite was true of uterine cancer. The latter cases were most likely to have been predominantly cervical cancer.

A similar considerable excess of female over male cancers of around three to one was also recorded in Paris and Geneva during the same period as the Verona study and in England and Wales between 1837 and 1842. Details of cancer subtypes in men and women at the Middlesex Hospital in the middle of the nineteenth century reveal a marked predominance of breast and uterine cancers, no mention of prostate cancer, and a modest though significant number of cancers in men that might be ascribed to smoking (these include lip, mouth, and tongue cancers, but very few lung cancers – cigarettes had yet to replace the pipe).

Unfortunately, these data still leave us unable to gauge accurately age-related incidence rates of common cancers in any society prior to the twentieth century. It is also important to distinguish between different subtypes of cancer that dramatically differ in incidence between different societies and are likely to have done so in the past. Several types of cancer have certainly been relatively common for many centuries, if not thousands of years. Overall, however, the prevalence of most of the current major cancers in Europe and North America, and especially lung cancer, was probably considerably lower prior to the twentieth century. At the same time, the apparent lower incidence of clinically recognized cancer in the seventeenth to nineteenth centuries may have numerous explanations – many individuals with incipient cancer will have succumbed to pre-emptive infectious deaths; diagnosis was imprecise and unaudited; and there was a likely failure to recognize some types of cancer, including perhaps prostatic cancers. Leukaemia was not diagnosed until 1845, by John Hughes Bennett in Edinburgh, but it's highly likely that cases existed for some time before this in line with the related cancer, lymphoma, which produces easily recognizable lumps and bumps.

Despite the lack of diagnostic ascertainment and statistics before and during the first half of the twentieth-century, it is clear that several cancers have increased in incidence during the last century and particularly in the last 50 years. A striking exception to this is stomach cancer. Gastric carcinomas have a very long and worldwide track record of trouble mongering. They were recognized by Hippocrates and Galen and detailed descriptions were provided by a fifteenth-century morbid anatomist in Florence, Antonio Benivieni. By the late nineteenth century, stomach cancer was recorded by Virchow as the most common cancer of men and a hundred years ago, in the USA, it was top of the cancer mortality stakes. And, although accurate figures are not available, it is highly likely that it was similarly the predominant cancer, at least in men, in Japan, China, other parts of South East Asia, and India, probably for many hundreds of years. Over the past sixty years incidence rates have declined dramatically in the West; much less so in other countries, including Japan, Chile, and China where stomach cancer remains in pole position, though soon to be overtaken by tobacco-related cancers.

Lung cancer linked to cigarette smoking and inhalation of the DNA-damaging combustion products of tobacco remains the one unambiguous example of a twentieth-century epidemic of cancer. It constitutes, along with other tobacco-related cancers, around a third of all cancers in the West. Yet these are not 'industrial' in the normal sense in which this term is used. Certainly the high incidence of these cancers is connected with commercial, manufacturing activities but this has to do not with the technical concoction of new poisons but rather facilitating access to, and delivery of, a natural, addictive carcinogenic cocktail. Even in this least ambiguous of cases, there is a long historical pedigree extending over centuries, including the eighteenth-century precedents of oral (lip, tongue, mouth, throat) cancer and pipe smoking, as well as factors other than just ignited tobacco itself, that tangibly contribute to risk. I deal with this very instructive tale of human fallibility in a later chapter.

Ironically, given the paucity of lung cancer in medical records prior to the twentieth century, it is one form of lung cancer, and one not connected with tobacco, that provides us with the earliest example of 'industrial' cancer. This is the persistent, if local, epidemic of lung cancer in uranium miners in the Erzgebirge or Ore Mountains around Schneeberg in what was part of Eastern Germany. Mining and occupational lung cancer can be traced back there for more than 500 years. The invisible mechanism – inhalation of a natural substance, DNA-damaging radon gas – was only identified much later.

And it is occupational cancer à la radon and sooty sweeps or environmental exposure to the pollutant waste products of petrochemical industrials that some regard as the hallmark of 'modern' cancers. With the recognition early in the twentieth century that chemical constituents of fired fossil fuels and other chemical products of industrial activity were carcinogenic, particularly for the skin, a mind-set developed that regarded man-made, concocted, or enriched chemical substances as the major agents in cancer – fuel for an epidemic. This view was projected to a crescendo in the late 1960s and 1970s as the environmentalists, inspired by Rachel Carson, politicians, and some scientists, with Chicago's Dr Samuel Epstein as their champion, developed and embellished the thesis that the apparent surge in cancer incidence, at least in the USA, was caused predominantly by a macho chemical industry and wanton pollution of the environment. (For pollution read petrochemical-based industrial waste effluents and pesticides in the water we drink, the air we breathe, and the food we eat.) Man-made radiation was added as an extra malevolent ingredient in the environmental pollution cocktail largely as a result of the cancerous consequences of the atomic bombs dropped on Japan in 1945. Tests of a small fraction of synthetic chemical products revealed that they could indeed be carcinogenic in rodents or mutate genes in bacteria (at very high doses), seemingly reinforcing the thesis.

We've moved on apace. No longer does melancholic predisposition lie at the heart of causation. A new bipartite game of noxious villains and passive victims was established in which the villain is money-grabbing capitalism and its techno-chemistry. Attempts to apportion a major share of cancer causation to lifestyle factors over which we might exercise some individual choice and control were emotively branded as 'blaming the victim'. The debate became extremely polarized and pugilistic. In the blue corner, weighing in with some force came Edith Efron. In her aptly entitled book *Apocalyptics*, she claimed that the environmentalist central idea lacked adequate or consistent evidence, was propelled by political and ideological agendas, and conveniently ignored the extraordinary wealth of potentially mutagenic and carcinogenic chemicals that exist naturally. In this latter respect, Bruce Ames took centre stage with virtuoso renditions on the theme of nature's natural carcinogenicity: mushrooms, broccoli, and wine were described as being richer in chemicals that could cause cancer (when given in very large doses to rodents) than environmental pollutants. The environmental pollution thesis was also underpinned by serious misinterpretation; the USA cancer science establishment at the National Cancer Institute made (mostly anonymous) pronouncements on cancer causes being 90 per cent 'environmental' which were widely misread as meaning synthetic chemicals plus man-made radiation. This was not what was meant and hard-nosed critics had to struggle to readjust the focus. As Robert Proctor superbly chronicled in his book *The Cancer Wars*, this whole debate or fight was, and still is, conducted in an arena where politics, ideology, and dogma are at best thinly veiled and reliable data on risks hard to come by.

The distinguished epidemiologists Richard Peto and Richard Doll have concluded that no more than 5 per cent of cancer deaths in the USA could be ascribed to exposure to products of our advanced technology (excluding cigarette manufacture) – not that 5 per cent represents a trivial or tolerable level. I'm not convinced anyone knows what the actual contribution of synthetic chemicals to the overall cancer burden is since the epidemiological study of this issue is excruciatingly difficult and negation of the hypothesis probably impossible. I suspect Peto and Doll are much nearer the mark than those activists and scientists who portray man-made environmental pollutants as the major players in a twentieth-century epidemic. It is unfortunate to say the least that views on this important issue are often highly charged, polarized, and evangelically pursued. There is a case to answer.

It seems to me reasonable to conclude that a small but significant minority of cancers are directly attributable to industrial activities or chemical products of our advanced technology in both developed and developing countries. However, there is little doubt that the majority of cancers do not originate from this source. Some cancers, notably those of the liver, oropharynx, oesophagus, and cervix are considerably more common in developing countries including China, South East Asia, parts of Latin America, and Africa. And around one half of the eight million plus cancers diagnosed each year occur in these less privileged settings.

Nevertheless, the current high rate of some types of cancer (breast, prostate, colon, and melanoma for example) in developed countries is in a sense attributable to industrialization or 'development' of society. But perhaps not for the usually presumed reason. Industrialization created crowded urban slums and facilitated endemic infections or epidemics which, combined with malnutrition, took a major toll on life, especially of infants and the elderly. Intense political pressure for social reforms during the latter part of the nineteenth century helped introduce improved sanitation and cleaner water which substantially reduced mortality before there was any real understanding of microbial hazards[6]. Only later, science came on the scene to further clean up with drugs and vaccination.

These dramatic changes in the health of industrialized nations greatly improved life expectancy but they had another quite unanticipated and paradoxical impact – on cancer incidence in both the very young and old. By greatly reducing the number of competing causes of death, a healthier society was now at increased risk of cancer – and not just because people were living longer. Industrial development in the West led eventually to a much more affluent, commercialized society and with it, dramatic changes in lifestyle, diet, and patterns of reproduction. These attributes of material progress provide the paradoxical context within which rates of some types of cancer can escalate whilst others decline. As we shall see.

So, cancer is emphatically not a new disease. It is endemic in the natural world and has been present in all human societies, albeit in differing forms and incidence rates. There has not been, is not, and probably will not ever be, a cancer-free Utopia. Patterns of cancer incidence change and they are in some essential way, with other illnesses, linked to cultural or social variation. Epidemiological sleuthing can help identify exposures and behavioural patterns that may be implicated in cancer aetiology. But understanding the causal mechanisms involved and the real why and how it happens is only possible with some biological archaeology – digging out what makes us tick, the deep legacies inherent in our design, and the pitfalls that can open the door to cancer.

CHAPTER 4

AN EVOLUTIONARY VIEW

Nothing in biology makes sense except in the light of evolution.

(Th. Dobzhansky, 1937)

What then is cancer? The answer you may get depends on what you want to know and how you pose the question. Some of the most vivid and moving descriptions of cancer have come from patients who happen to be writers or journalists.[7] These accounts portray what cancer is, in terms of personal impact, uncertainty, and pain: an insider's story. If, on the other hand, you are looking for details of different cancers, gene mutations or of hazards to avoid, tests to take, or available treatments and averaged outcomes, then these data are available in your library or on internet web sites. This information contributes to the overall picture but does not in itself constitute either an explanation of why we get cancer or an adequate prescription for what makes a cancer. I'm aiming for something different.

A major difficulty here is how to draw a multidimensional and dynamic picture in which essential details highlight principles rather than obfuscate. Another challenge is to incorporate the diversity of cancer plus the pervasive role of chance without portraying the process as inaccessible chaos. The problem is largely one of diversity, dimensions, and vocabulary. The focus of action spans the smallest subunit-nucleotide bases in DNA, to cells, to whole bodies; it encompasses human history and social behaviour; and it occupies time frames from hours to decades to millions of years. The language normally used to illuminate these various parameters differs and is not generally exportable across the boundaries.

An explanation is required within which the variable time frames, components, and capricious characteristics of cancer can be comfortably accommodated. An explanation not only of the mechanics of how cancer happens and of the therapeutically intransigent nature of the illness but also of the broader conundrum of why. The role of chance must make sense rather than being a shield for our ignorance.

It is my view that the perspective that best explains cancer is a Darwinian, evolutionary picture. By best, I mean quite simply that it works better for me than anything else that I am aware of. Works in the sense of both accommodating most of the established, diverse facts about cancer and also provides plausible explanations for the major puzzles. Why does a healthy body get cancer? Why is there so much of it about and why are different types of cancers predominant in different countries? Why do so many things appear to cause cancer? Why does it often take decades to emerge? Why does treatment sometimes succeed but more usually fail? Is it just bad luck and why me? Or, why not me?

The essential idea is tried and tested. It is *the* central unifying theme of biology and is being increasingly recognized as contributing to our better understanding of the human condition in health and disease. H C Trowell and D P Burkitt, physician and surgeon respectively, with lengthy experience of working in East Africa, had astutely observed the changing trends in the incidence of cancer and other 'Western' modern diseases as black African populations became urbanized and adopted some of the lifestyle characteristics of Europeans. They saw this medical dilemma as a paradoxical price of 'progress', the penalties reflecting an impact of rapid social and environmental change on communities long adapted for a very different lifestyle, particularly with respect to diet and physical activity. This interpretation of common chronic diseases has been given the apt descriptive label of evolutionary or Darwinian medicine by Randolph Nesse and George Williams. What they (along with S Boyd Eaton, W M S Russell, and other protagonists) have sought to portray is an historical and evolutionary perspective on why our bodies are vulnerable to particular diseases.[8] Evolutionary biology can show how disorders that are particularly prevalent in human societies can be usefully viewed, not just in terms of proximate or immediate causes, but as a consequence of discord between our inherent genetics, anatomy, and physiology and our rapid acquisition of novel diets and lifestyles. This promises to give us a new and valuable perspective on medical problems as diverse as obesity, diabetes, heart disease, skeletal and joint degeneration, pregnancy complications, myopia, and many aspects of ageing. The evolutionary dimension is also essential to any understanding of the emergence of infectious micro-organisms and their disease correlates. There is little doubt that evolutionary biology can similarly help explain why we get cancer and the preponderance of different cancers in human societies at different times, and why we now seem to be in such a mess.

The starting premise in this narrative on cancer is that the proximal or immediate cause is variation or mutation in genes, a game of chance played out by rules both constrained and liberated by our evolutionary history. Mutant genes and the clones of cells in which they reside, take centre stage in this story. This is a necessary though not in itself sufficient condition for a credible explanation. The larger picture of causation is altogether richer, multidimensional, and more interesting. Here are the three evolutionary ingredients of the story to follow, provided as a taster or synopsis.

(1) The penalty clauses

Cancer reflects intrinsic penalty clauses in our evolutionary history. Two are of very ancient origin. The first is the imperfect fidelity of DNA copying, management and repair from which follows an intrinsic mutability of our genes. The genetic code isn't sacrosanct; indeed if it were, evolution itself would not be possible. A certain level of error proneness is an evolutionary necessity. Moreover, genes are not vacuum sealed on chromosomes but are inevitably exposed to a hostile world. Life has evolved on a planet that has a naturally radioactive geology and that is bathed in a solar and cosmic source of electro-magnetic radiation. A narrow spectrum of this we register as visible light and heat but other terrestrial and extraterrestrial rays are cryptic to our senses. Those with ionizing activity, such as gamma rays, can, by energy transfer, impart charge (or ionize) and alter the structure of water molecules and DNA in cells. Or, in the case of UVB, rays may interact with and change the conformation of DNA in exposed cells. In other words they can be mutagenic. The biosphere itself creates, without the exigencies of man, a wealth of toxins, poisons, pesticides, chemicals, and infectious agents that can directly or indirectly damage or mutate DNA if present or consumed in high enough concentrations.

To this external assault, add the endogenous chemistry of our bodies. Our tissue physiology and cellular metabolism is oxygen-fuelled and, paradoxical as it may sound, by-products of this process can and do damage DNA. These natural and ubiquitous exposures make a contribution to what is sometimes called spontaneous mutation and might even, with ionizing radiation for example, have placed planet Earth at an early evolutionary advantage as far as an emerging biology was concerned. Mutations happen all the time and are blind to consequences. This is the base upon which natural selection and evolution operates in nature.

The second advantageous but inherently dangerous legacy is a physiological requirement, especially in more complex multicellular creatures including ourselves, for cellular functions that endow resilience but are pregnant with malignant potential: the phenotypic plasticity and extensive proliferation capacity of certain cells, coupled with mobility and invasive ability, plus the availability of lymphatic and vascular channels for cell migration. These quasi-cancerous properties are essential features of embryo development, inflammation and wound healing, tissue renewal, stress responses, and placental function in pregnancy. They reflect a well-orchestrated exploitation of a billion-year-old genetic memory of cells to survive stress, clone, and expand their territory. Genes subserving these essential functions are mostly of very ancient evolutionary origin. And, as part of our gene pool, they too can be subject to the mutational lottery. There is therefore an inherent potential risk of mutation and cancer in our genetic and physiological make-up – unavoidable historical baggage.

At the same time however, there has been evolutionary pressure for the development of restraints on mutation and cancerous cell behaviour. These have been necessary not only to reduce the potential impact of cancer on reproductive fitness but also act more immediately to ensure social cohesiveness of cellular activity without which embryos could never achieve their architecturally demanding objective and there would be no resilience of tissue function. Diets contain, or should contain (mostly from plant sources), minerals, vitamins, and a variety of other chemicals that have protective or antioxidant properties. We are also very well endowed with genes encoding protein products that have restraining or caretaker roles, including detection and repair of damaged DNA, detoxification, and antioxidant function.

Other controls exercise jurisdiction over the aspirations of single cells to go forth and multiply. Essential though this proclivity is, it has to be constrained in time and space. This is achieved both by the internal wiring of cells and by the social and structural organization of cells into interactive tissue compartments. Compulsive or persistent proliferation of cells can be registered within the cell as potentially disruptive and fail-safe mechanisms activated that compel the would-be escapees to adopt either an alternative lifestyle of slumbering quiescence or a suicidal demise. Physical liaisons between cells and networks of chemical signals oscillating throughout the tissue environments impose strict rules of residence and behaviour that normally ensure that expansionist tendencies are only transiently expressed. Penalties for transgression can again be severe – cell death, for example.

These caretaker functions and social contracts within and between all cells in multicellular creatures, including ourselves, are legislated by genes, many of which are of very considerable evolutionary antiquity. Similar genes are found not only in invertebrate species but, in some cases, in yeast, unicellular organisms, and even bacteria. Moreover, such genes tend to be remarkably preserved in evolution, to the extent that not only do human genes exercising these functions have recognizably similar coding sequences to their equivalents in yeast but they can carry out their prescribed function when engineered into yeast.

Generally speaking, a billion (1000 million)-year-old ancestry and conserved structure/function indicates cell activity that empowered survival or reproductive success and was rewarded with the stamp of adaptive approval – an open-ended evolutionary licence to practise. Without these surveillance and mopping-up operations, life as we know it probably could not exist. But they are not omnipotent and the trade-off is that these controls minimize but cannot eliminate the occurrence of mutations in DNA. And then of course these regulatory genes too cannot be immune to mutation.

The resultant genetic game of chance has been loaded heavily in favour of survival. Still, our tissues have been structured to oscillate on the edge of chaos and the scales can be tipped the wrong way by exposure of cells and tissues to chronic or persistent stress, naturally occurring environmental or endogenous chemicals that damage DNA, and by chance mutation. As a consequence, small tumours and a modest level of cancers are inevitable and widespread in nature.[9] And we are all poised closer to the precipice than we might like to imagine.

(2) The social ratchet

Homo sapiens occupy a special and unenviable place in this scheme of things. Superimposed on our very ancient genetic memories is a more recent, million-year-old evolutionary legacy that we acquired or modified as an emerging species of hominid primates. This inheritance lays down, in the language of DNA, our own game plan for reproductive fitness coupled with an extraordinary capacity for social engineering. But it is flawed as far as cancer is concerned. Flawed by a double whammy from what were, originally, very advantageous adaptations. First, our ability to survive long after our natural reproductive period. Second, our propensity to interfere with both our own and other people's biology. Examples include our persistent pursuit of pleasure in the form of smoking, sunshine, and sex and, rather less transparently, our adoption of diets, physical inactivity, and reproductive patterns that are at odds with our inherent biology. The undesirable biological consequences are slow, chronic, and stealth-like, impacting mostly after our normal reproductive period. They escape the evolutionary filter of natural selection and conspire together to both outflank and exploit the efficacy of otherwise very resilient biological controls.

We have become social beasts out of synch with our genetics, caught in a nature-nurture mismatch, our pedestrian genetics too slow to catch up with or adapt to our strident and exotic social habits. The consequence is accumulative damage and a potent ratcheting-up of risk for the emergence of cancer in an ageing and puzzled body. But the 'indecent' exposures involved are not unitary, omnipotent, or exclusive causes; they form part of a composite network of socially engineered risk attributes that may have long, variable, and complex historical origins that filter into a common underlying biological mechanism. And that mechanism is itself remarkably Darwinian in its operation.

(3) The dominant clone

Despite the risks imposed by our genetic history when coupled with our lifestyle, of all the billions of cells produced in our bodies each day, it is usually just one cell and its descendant clone that breaks through in a lifetime to cause havoc. Stringent restraints face compounded risks in a prolonged confrontation and chance then has the final say. The issue isn't just why do we get cancer but why not? The explanation for this conundrum lies in the extraordinary way in which cancer develops or evolves. The biological process of cancer development, initiated by DNA mishaps and leading to a territorially dominant clone, turns out to be a remarkable parody of species diversification in evolution. It operates on a micro-scale and embodies the essential Darwinian ground rules of random genetic diversification and clonal selection for survival and reproductive advantage in novel territories or ecosystems. But this isn't just a parallel with evolution, it is evolution – in cells with a 2000-million-year-old genetic memory of unicellular selfishness. Our cells are latent parasites and can become so – the ultimate in atavism.

Identical twins (and Dolly) have acquainted us with the notion of clones as genetically identical copies. The paradox in cancer is that although each cancer is a clone, it is the *lack* of genetic uniformity that is the key to its imperialistic success. Cancer clones evolve and diversify, over variable but usually very protracted periods of years and decades, by sequential addition of mutations in different genes that collectively corrupt cell behaviour. These then provide a genetic passport through the major evolutionary bottlenecks: the initial formation of a tumour; next, tumour to cancer transition with spread within tissues followed by dissemination or metastasis to other tissues; and then, finally, survival of the decimation elicited by therapy. This process involves exceedingly rare or chance events; each key mutational step empowering a single cell and its descendants. For such a process to generate cells with a genetic 'full house' of aberrations takes a long time and the odds are so heavily stacked against, that very few cells, of the millions with aspirations, can acquire fully-fledged cancerous credentials. The winning cellular phenotypes are very rare, the drop-out rate is huge, but the culmination of this process is a mutinous species of cell or clone that has shut off the safety valves of differentiation and death, and reproduces itself continually as an immortal clone with territorial dominance of the body habitat. An ancient past revisited but, critically, in a closed and fragile ecosystem. In an evolutionary time frame, this is certainly fast track, but from an individual patient's perspective it is not, except towards the end as clonal dominance may escalate in its pathological impact. The extended time frame required for the clonal evolution of cancer and the lack of a simple or linear relationship between cause and outcome are crucial features that both frustrate the unambiguous identification of risks and temper the acceptance of known risks.

Uncovering the genetic circuits disrupted or uncoupled by mutation has revealed the molecular and biochemical mechanisms that drive the Darwinian development of cancer clones and provides a highly plausible explanation of why so many factors can contribute directly or indirectly, singly and in combination, to cancer causation. It has, at the same time, produced unexpected and profound insights into basic biological processes of cell life and death. Perhaps most crucially of all, in practical terms, these molecular details identify potential Achilles' heels for cancer cells and provide a route map to new diagnostic and therapeutic strategies. At the same time they have revealed why conventional therapy is likely to be frustrated once cancer has gained a foothold. It wasn't exactly the answer cancer physicians and pharmacologists had been anticipating and which had been used as a rationale for therapeutic design.

In all these evolutionary components of cancer, chance is the joker in the pack. Chance operates at every level in the multidimensional causal pathway of cancer, as indeed it does in biological evolution in general – not least for us in the genetic lottery that operates at the moment of conception. Our individually unique inherited gene set (a mixed parental legacy tarnished, in some cases, with cancer gene mutations) distorts the odds for cancer, as it does for most other diseases, as well as for more desirable attributes. But the odds can be shifted – if you know how the game is played.

NOTES TO PART ONE

1 And is in good company with many scientists who can be blinkered or parochial when it comes to understanding causal pathways. See critique by Steven Rose (1997) *Lifelines*, Penguin Press, London.

2 Picture of Ferrante I of Arragon (aged 40–50 years) taken from 'Adorazione dei Magi' by M Cardisco. Kindly provided by Drs A Marchetti and G Fornaciari. Descriptions of his tumour are provided in: Fornaciari G (1994) *Journal of the History of Medicine*, **6**:139–46; Marchetti A *et al.* (1996) *Lancet*, **347**:1272.

3 Don Brothwell from the British Natural History Museum, along with other palaeopathologists, has made extensive studies of such remains. Brothwell DR and Sandison AT (1967) *Diseases in antiquity*, Charles Thomas Publishers, Illinois.

4 Good reviews of the early history of cancer medicine are in: Haagenson CD (1933) An exhibit of important books, papers and memorabilia illustrating the evolution of knowledge of cancer, *Am J Cancer*, **18**:42–146; De Moulin D (1983) *A short history of breast cancer*, Kluwers Academic Publishers, Dordrecht.

5 Much of Hunter's writings on cancer were, allegedly, plagiarized by his brother-in-law, Evarard Home, who also had the temerity to burn Hunter's manuscripts. Cohen B (1993) John Hunter Pathologist, *J Royal Soc Med*, **86**:587–92; Robson J (1959) John Hunter's views on cancer, *Ann Royal Coll Surg Engl*, **25**:176–81.

6 See Dubois R (1959) *Mirage of health. Utopias, progress and biological change*. Harpers Brothers Publishing, New York.

7 There are many such books to commend but the best for me were: Diamond J (1998) *C because cowards get cancer too*, Vermilion Publishing, London; and Picardie R (1998) *Before I say goodbye*, Penguin Books, London. Other authors have used their personal experiences with cancer as a platform to explore or advocate a particular view on causation. Ecologist and Rachel Carson devotée, Sandra Steingraber's *Living downstream* (1988, Virago Books) is one of the best crafted of these.

8 A good summary of these early insights into cancer through the eyes of evolutionary medicine is in: Trowell HC and Burkitt DP (1981) *Western*

diseases: their emergence and prevention, Edward Arnold Publishers, London. For later, more comprehensive analyses and insights into evolutionary or Darwinian medicine, see the following: Nesse RM and Williams GC (1995) *Evolution and healing. The new science of Darwinian medicine*, Weidenfeld and Nicolson (originally published in the USA in 1994 by Times Books as *Why we get sick*); Nesse RM and Williams GC (1998) Evolution and the origins of disease, *Scientific American*, **November**:58–65; Stearns SC, ed. (1999) *Evolution in health and disease*, Oxford University Press, Oxford, for a collection of excellent reviews. See also Paul Ewald, ed. (1994) *Evolution of infectious diseases*, Oxford University Press, Oxford.

9   For a review of tumours and cancer in other animals, as well as plants, see Becker FF, ed. (1975) *Cancer*, Vol 4, Plenum Press, New York.

FURTHER READING

Ames B and Gold LS (1989) Pesticides, risks and apple sauce. *Science*, **244**:755–7.

Ames BN, Profet M, Gold LS (1990) Nature's chemicals and synthetic chemicals: comparative toxicology. *Proc Natl Acad Sci USA*, **87**:7782–6.

Doll R and Peto R (1981) *The causes of cancer*. Oxford University Press, Oxford.

Efron E (1984) *The apocalyptics: cancer and the big lie – how environmental politics controls what we know about cancer*. Simon and Schuster, New York.

Epstein SS (1979) *The politics of cancers*. Anchor Press, New York.

Greer S (1983) Cancer and the mind. *Br J Psychiat*, **143**:535–43.

Kowal, SJ (1955) Emotions as a cause of cancer. *The Psychoanalytic Review*, **42**:217–27.

Proctor R (1995) *Cancer wars*. Basic Books, New York.

Roberts C and Manchester K (1995) *The archaeology of disease*. 2nd edn. Cornell University Press.

Rothschild BM, Witzke BJ, Schultz M (1999) Metastatic cancer in the Jurassic. *Lancet*, **354**:398.

Satinoff MI and Wells C (1969) Multiple basal cell naevus syndrome in ancient Egypt. *Med History*, **13**: 294–7.

Shimkin MB (1977) *Contrary to nature – cancer*. US Department of Health, Education and Welfare. Public Health Service, NIH, USA.

Sontag S (1983) *Illness as metaphor*. Penguin Books.

Stathopolous G (1975) Kanam mandible tumour. *Lancet*, **I**:165.

Walshe WH (1846) *Nature and the treatment of cancer.* (Includes presentation of Rigoni-Stern's data on cancer incidence in Verona.) Taylor and Walton, London.

PART TWO

EVOLVING CANCER

The overall picture of the natural history of cancer, once it has been
initiated, is characteristically Darwinian.

(MacFarlane Burnet, 1974)

What has been learned from oncogenes represents the first peep behind
the curtain that for so long has obscured the mechanisms of
cancer. In one respect, the first look is unnerving, because the
chemical mechanisms that seem to drive the cancer cell astray are not
different in kind from mechanisms at work in the normal cell.

(Michael Bishop, 1982)

Selection [in evolution] has no eyes for the future.

(George Williams, 1966)

CHAPTER 5

PUNDIT'S PROGRESS

Our attempt to understand the essential nature of cancer has been a long, drawn-out process. Progress has been in part a slow progression, part dormancy, but then with periodic leaps empowered by technical advances in surgery, microscopy, pathology, and genetics.

The ancient Greeks and Romans recognized several types of cancers but many of their vague and erroneous ideas persisted unchallenged for 1500 years and more. For almost two millennia, cancer, as a medical problem, lay almost exclusively within the domain of surgeons and pathologists. This explains why societies prohibiting or eschewing these disciplines in medical training, such as the Chinese and most of Europe during the Dark Ages, made little or no progress in identifying and treating cancer. In medieval Europe, medical acumen with regard to cancer lay with Islamic surgeons and physicians practising throughout the Mediterranean region from Baghdad to Cordoba.

Not that any society, 'Western' or otherwise, made much progress. Opinions of learned men were constrained, not just by knowledge and technical limitations, but by philosophical doctrines of the day. The ancient Babylonian and Greek thesis of the universality of the four elements (air, water, fire, and earth) and their analogous humours in the body (blood, phlegm, yellow bile, and black bile) proved a mental gridlock. This finds a parallel in Oriental societies where traditional medicine interpreted for centuries, and to some extent still does today, tumorous growths as imbalances in the forces of nature that pervade the universe – the Yin and Yang and the five elements. We will eventually need a holistic view of the cancer problem but there are, unfortunately, no short cuts.

The equivalent of a Copernican revision in cancer medicine was in abeyance until the Renaissance provided the philosophical and intellectual climate for a new beginning. This required insight into our anatomical and cellular structure and began with the discovery of the circulatory system of blood by William Harvey and later of the lymphatics by Gaspare Aselli in Milano. A Parisian surgeon, Henri François Le Dran, published a memoir in 1757 for which he is credited with the first clear recognition that cancer starts off as a small local lesion but then spreads via the lymphatics to local lymph nodes. Later, in 1829, Récamier described invasion of breast cancer cells into veins and coined the term 'metastasis' for the more distant spread of cancer cells, for example from the breast to the brain. Those advances owed a great deal to the invention and technical elaboration of the microscope. This also led to the recognition, especially by Theodor Schwann and then Rudolf Virchow and the German school in the nineteenth century, of the fundamental role of the cell in pathology. By the mid-nineteenth century, the cellular interpretation of normal tissue architecture and its disruption in diseases including cancer was well recognized. Wilhem Waldeyer in particular laid the foundation of much of our current views of cancer by suggesting that it arose by the transformation of individual normal cells into malignant cells by external factors, followed by local, then widespread, dissemination via either lymph or blood.

These advances substantially improved knowledge of cancer at a descriptive level but provided no real insight into underlying mechanisms. This required Watson and Crick to unlock the genetic code in DNA – but even this crucial leap forward has important antecedents. At the beginning of this century, Theodor Boveri, a remarkably talented German embryologist, predicted that cancer originated in single cells as a consequence of changes or imbalances in genetic information which his experiments on sea urchin embryos led him to believe must reside in the chromosomes of cells. This suggestion, entirely novel at the time, was not well received but has turned out to be extraordinarily prescient. Other experimental studies in the twentieth century, but well before the modern molecular era, had a major impact on our understanding of the biological mechanisms underlying cancer. Ernest Kennaway and his colleagues, working at the Institute of Cancer Research in London in the 1920s, were able to isolate the polycyclic hydrocarbons responsible for the cancer-causing properties of coal tars – the first carcinogens to be identified. Later, in the 1960s, in a landmark study at the same Institute, Brookes and Lawley discovered that carcinogenic chemicals react directly with the genetic material (DNA) rather than, as others had suspected, ribonucleic acid or protein. This finding was then a crucial precursor to mutational explanations for cancer as was Hermann Muller's observation in the late 1920s that ionizing radiation mutated DNA.

In cancer research however, as in most areas of biology and medicine, the turning point really was the decoding of DNA itself by Watson and Crick in 1953. Pandora's box was opened and the ramifications have been extra-ordinary. This made possible the modern era of cancer molecular biology whose dazzling pace in unravelling fundamental mechanisms has been well charted by Weinberg, Varmus, Bishop, and other major players in the game. It may seem mean spirited not to re-navigate this recent history for readers but this has been done already and I would rather distil from it what important ideas and principles have emerged and, in particular, how the molecular details can be interpreted within an evolutionary framework.

CHAPTER 6

CLONES, CLONES, CLONES

If there is one respect in which cancer is special as an illness, it is that all the cancer cells in one patient are, in almost every case, derived from a single cell. They are a clone. Not necessarily all identical because the capacity of the progeny of the founder or mother cell to diversify genetically is another critical feature of cancer cells, as we shall see – but a clone nonetheless. A clone of up to or more than 10^{12} (a million, million) cells that may have dispersed throughout the body. A clone that if removed from the confines of the body could, given suitable conditions, expand to fill any large and well-known building. But clones – multiple copies of the same thing, abound in nature.

Charles Darwin introduced the idea of common descent, by which he meant that, historically, every group of organisms is descendent from a common single ancestor and that collectively all forms of life can be backtracked to a single origin. Evolution is clonal at its core. All asexually reproducing organisms, including bacteria, viruses, fungi, and some more complex plant and animal species propagate as clones. All the dandelions plaguing your lawn and all the aphids terrorizing your rose beds may well belong to single clones. Recently some hitherto unrecognized fern-like conifer trees were discovered in Australia's Wollemi National Park. This ancient species, now named *Wollemia nobilis*, dates back 300 million years and as individual specimens appear to be genetically identical, they are probably the members of a single and remarkably stable clone. As the progeny of a clone disseminate geographically, we lose sight of their potential or actual size and biomass. In rare instances clonal descendants stick together and the result can be impressive, as in the case of a giant fungus that covers around 15 hectares of forest soil in Montana.

The outgrowth of an antibiotic-resistant strain of bacteria or DDT-resistant insects is often (though not always) a clonal phenomenon: emergence of a dominant clone derived from a single mutant individual generated by random diversification in DNA but with selective survival advantage in the presence of a lethal chemical assault. The generation of a novel infectious virus, such as HIV, is probably the clonal product of one unique virus, as are many epidemics of both common and exotic infections. Periodic influenza epidemics may arise via the novel infectious properties or immunological invisibility of a new mutant or clonal variety of the virus. Recent epidemics of drug-resistant tuberculosis (*Mycobacterium tuberculosis*) in the 1990s in New York and of streptococcus (*S. pyogenes*) with infectious complications including rheumatic fever and toxic shock syndrome in the late 1980s have both been mapped by genetic fingerprinting to unique or clonal strains of bacteria. Even parasites derived from species that normally reproduce sexually may find advantage by propagating asexually as mutant clones.[1]

Identical twins are members of the one natural human clone – derived from the same single fertilized egg. Man has been artificially cloning offspring for a long time before Dolly the sheep, the genetic offspring of a single adult mammary gland cell, came along to stir up our emotions. Agriculturists have been cloning bananas, sweet potatoes, date palms, and vines from selected seeds and grafts for centuries and probably for millennia. Commercial viniculture has been dependent upon the ease of cloning plants. There are whole vineyards, and forests, that are clonal in origin. In these examples, replicates are formed by binary fission of cells. It works in nature because the genetic code (DNA) can be copied and doubled up prior to division in order to provide each offspring cell with the same genetic information and the template for further copies. The most basic property of biological systems throughout evolution has been their propensity to clone. Cloning is expansion by non-sexual reproduction. Expansion increases chances of survival. Playing by numbers.

Cloning coupled with Darwinian or natural selection also goes on in our bodies, all the time. For starters, all the cells of our body are members of a single clone, derived that is from a single cell (the fertilized egg). The reason we don't all look like slime moulds is that we have lots of specialized subclones within the master clone. The clearest example of cloning within our bodies is however with the immune system. Here we have a really neat trick that was first adopted by one of our jawed vertebrate ancestors some 450 million years ago. This operates on the basis of clonal cell generation and natural selection. Lymphocytes are generated continuously in the bone marrow and thymus and undergo a remarkable process of gene shuffling. From a basic building block of around a hundred genes encoding the sequence information for making an antibody protein, some tens of millions of antibody gene sets are generated. The shuffling process is choreographed in such a way that once a cell has one rearranged, functional antibody gene, this is inherited by all clonal descendants. Each of these unique antibodies can identify or bind to any complementary molecular shapes – or antigens – in a lock-and-key fashion, and then solicit appropriate cellular responses.

The process of clonal diversification is essentially random or blind to specific utility; anticipatory and catch-all. Antibody cells are primed to recognize any one of a million or more foreign 'shapes' that might, or might not, come along as the flags of microbial invasion. Lymphocyte clones, that coincidentally recognize self-structures in our own bodies, are mostly eliminated or inhibited from expanding. In contrast, following infection, individual clones, from one to a few hundred, recognize alien shapes and respond by selectively proliferating to provide a protective immune response. The proliferative potential of the selected clones and resultant clone size can be very impressive (many millions of cells), as can the longevity of such clones (over decades or even a human life span).

The immune system might appear to be unique in the selective expansion of genetically diverse clones, by Darwinian selection that is. But it isn't entirely. In any one individual or multicellular animal, all normal cells will have the same DNA and set of genes, with the exception of the polydiverse immune cells and red blood cells that are DNA-less. The formation of a normal offspring from the nucleus of a sheep mammary cell is a dramatic proof of this point. Clones of cells within an individual can be functionally distinct however by having a different and stable pattern of selective gene expression – a different song to sing from the same extensive genetic repertoire. This involves changes in the higher order structure of DNA on chromosomes. All the information for the complete repertoire of the species is still there in every cell but is now regulated so that only restricted components can function in any one cell or clone of cells – a compartmentalized genotype. It's on this basis that multi-cellular organisms with specialized cells and tissues evolved in the first place. But a long-standing rule of this arrangement for a conglomerate of diverse clones is that you only sing when told to and you stick to the same few songs.

Exactly how a single fertilized egg generates a coherent pattern of cells, into tissues, organs, and structures whose individual songs are orchestrated into a symphony from one score is one of the major unresolved challenges of biology. But the picture is becoming clearer, thanks to the power of molecular biology. It turns out that the process is imbued with Darwinian principles of variation and natural selection. The process of embryogenesis by which our body plan is specified in the embryo involves survival and proliferation of small numbers of founder cells for different tissues – selective survival and clonal expansion, as opposed to death by default, for the modest number of cells that find them-selves in the right place at the right time and are either singing the right tune or can be induced to do so as an adaptation to their surroundings. As a con-sequence, our tissues are structured as a mosaic of clones with specialized function or genetic repertoire. Each crypt surrounding the protruding villi of the intestinal wall is formed as a single clone, as are tracks or zones of up to two million cells or 10 millimetres wide in bladder and breast ductal epithelium, brain tissue, arterial walls, and skin. Some neurobiologists, Gerald Edelman in particular, suspect that the establishment of neural networks and the extra-ordinary repertoire of the brain parallels the immune system and utilizes Darwinian selection. The model proposed involves the selective survival of cells or clusters of cells which form contacts and potential networks, and the subsequent fine-tuning or consolidation of networks via external stimuli.

Clonal junkies

Cellular clones can cause us big problems if they are allowed to proliferate and extend their territory. Immune clones can backfire and cause disease. If, for example, the alien shape of an infectious microbe just happens to resemble or mimic that of some internal molecule of our own bodies, autoreactive clones of immune cells (lymphocytes) may then expand and cause tissue damage. This is the likely scenario for multiple sclerosis, rheumatic fever, some forms of arthritis, and insulin-dependent diabetes. Clonal expansion in these situations may be perpetuated or re-established in the constant presence of the self-stimulating tissue antigens or following reinfection.

Atherosclerotic plaques, which develop in the arteries, are clonal growths too. The single-cell origin or monoclonality of plaques has puzzled cardiologists for the past two decades. These lesions reflect an excessive wound-healing response to chronic vascular injury and contribute to the only other major causes of death (strokes and myocardial infarction) in the Western world to compete with cancer. But why should the plaques derive from a single cell? Recent evidence indicates that the cells within such vascular lesions are mutants. Genetic instability in these cells may involve loss of activity in cell surface receptor molecules whose function is to receive negative signals restraining growth. Acquired insensitivity to such inhibitory signals would be functionally equivalent to drug resistance, providing any mutant clone with a selective growth advantage. How such mutations arise is unclear but oxidative stress from chronic inflammation and a mutagenic impact of cigarette smoking are possible causes. In effect, atherosclerotic plaques are mini-tumours.

Evolving through the bottlenecks

Cancer cells are then exercising a fundamental and ancient biological function – a two billion-year-old proclivity for clonal self-replication. How then are they different from other cells and why does it cause such havoc? They are, for a start, mutants; multiple mutants in fact. The cancer clone is assembled, piecemeal, and at each stage, subclones with novel behavioural properties emerge until a point of no return is reached. The cells acquire selective advantage because their accumulated sets of mutations progressively unleash a pattern of inherent primal properties: persistent cloning in the face of signals for restraint, immortality in stark rebuttal of normal cell death commands, and a capacity for territorial expansion beyond the confines of normal barriers and rules of residence. They behave as if they were blind, selfish, and atavistic. This is biological chaos – a pattern of cellular behaviour engendering progressive disorder in the context of normal tissue function as communication breaks down.[2]

The analogy between the development of cancer clones and the evolution of new species has been made many times in the past. However the new molecular discoveries in cancer research have greatly reinforced the validity and value of this comparison at the levels of cells and genes, to the extent that we can now see that cancer doesn't just parody evolution, it is a form of evolution played by the same Darwinian ground rules as apply to evolution in general and particularly for asexually propagating species. The essential game plan is progressive genetic diversification by mutation within a clone, coupled with selection of individual cells on the basis of reproductive and survival fitness, endorsed by their particular mutant gene set. It's evolution in the fast track.

All cancers arise or are initiated and then propelled by gene mutations in single cells. The initiating mutation is the lift-off point in cancer clone evolution, even though it may frequently be preceded by more global disturbances in tissue function affecting many cells. Cancer clones continuously evolve by genetic diversification and selection within each clone. Selective pressure derives from the physiological and physical constraints of the body and within the cancer cell itself. And following a diagnosis comes therapeutic intervention, providing potent selective pressure for survivors (cancer cells that is). Here we see a clear parallel with the evolution of parasites and the development of drug resistance in pathogenic organisms. Subclones of cancer cells and normal cells, in essence, compete for dominance of the body habitat. This confrontation is almost entirely covert (clinically speaking), takes multiple directions, and can wax and wane. In a minority of such skirmishes, a point of no return or take-off is reached as the gravitational pull of restraint is breached. The chronic and protracted natural history of the clone then culminates in a widespread territorial hijack. Clinically, this translates to pathological compromise of normal tissue function, high-grade malignancy, and, if unchallenged, in death.

But such catastrophes can have surprisingly innocuous beginnings. All cancers start off life as small and topographically confined clonal growths or mini-tumours and may acquire physical distinction as warts, polyps, fibromas, birthmarks, moles, or small tumours. Or they may be invisible as a discrete structure even under the microscope but detectable by molecular scrutiny as a mutated and clonally expanded patch of tissue. These are all very common and overwhelmingly benign or stalled in evolutionary progression to cancer. Leiomyoma tumours (uterine fibroids) are a pain in the uterine neck for many women and although they very rarely progress to malignancy, they provide a common reason for hysterectomy. Female Asian elephants and rhinos, as well as other non-human primates, have exactly the same problem – though they usually suffer in silence. The birthmark dark moles of Caucasian skin have for centuries been held as beauty marks or, for a while in the Middle Ages, as a signature of the devil – the one clonal growth or mini-tumour to acquire cult status. And they have been given religious significance too. The presence of moles on the upper body of a two-year-old child was an essential part of his qualification and incarnation as the fourteenth Dalai Lama in Tibet some 65 years ago.[3]

Leukaemias (blood cell cancers) have the same beginnings except that their clonal origin becomes diffused in the bone marrow or blood and is therefore never visible as a bump or a lump. We each and every one of us have many such clonal escapees and the vast majority remain benign, asymptomatic, or clinically silent, and may regress and disappear. They do however represent the seed-corn from which a dominant cancer clone can, over time, emerge. But then emergence and 'success' requires negotiation of some very significant hurdles. These are the evolutionary bottlenecks for cancer.

A major restraint or bottleneck in the natural history of most tumour to cancer transitions is the neovascularization or new blood vessel formation required for tumours to expand beyond a minimal size (around a hundred million cells or a volume of around one to two cubic millimetres). Failure of cells with an expansionist tendency to solicit an adequate blood supply results in oxygen deprivation and suffocation (of the tumour). Another, and possibly the most critical, bottleneck in cancer clones' uncertain journey is the physical set of boundaries within and between tissues that delineate cellular territory and impose rules of residential restraint. To escape beyond this locale, cancer cells must express the ability to degrade physical barriers, expand within tissues, emigrate, infiltrate, and colonize other tissue ecosystems. Emigration to new tissue sites, or metastasis, is the clinically critical transition point in cancer evolution.

The unnatural history following therapeutic intervention by the oncologist provides the final major evolutionary bottleneck for cancer cells involving widespread decimation and strong selective pressure for survival mutants. Very few cells make it through the bottlenecks.

The evolutionary development of cancer can be relatively rapid – for example, less than a year for some infant cancers that arise in rapidly pro-liferating and highly mobile cells in the foetus. But more commonly, in adults, its natural history spans very many years or several decades. This extended time frame largely reflects the low probability of single cells accumulating a set of mutations that can provide the passport and visas required to negotiate the bottlenecks. To understand how mutations in cancer cells can drive or release territorial expansion that is blind to its deleterious impact, we need to take an evolutionary look at how genes influence cell behaviour.

CHAPTER 7

THE WAY WE ARE: RISKS AND RESTRAINTS

In the antique but thriving world of unicellular life forms such as bacteria and many protozoa, as well as viruses, success is a transparent process of self-perpetuation – a numbers game. The evolution of multicellular organisms some 700 million years ago was a critical transition point engendering more sophisticated survival and reproductive strategies involving specialization of cells and tissues, coupled with interdependence of cells and subservience of the parts to the whole. But this co-operative form of life does not eliminate the capacity of constituent cells to proliferate as clones and, under some circumstances, to migrate across tissue boundaries, or to behave, at least temporarily, like unicellular organisms or cancer cells. Indeed, these are critical functions for embryo development, in tissue renewal, inflammation, wound healing, immunity, and, in mammals, pregnancy. Evolution has therefore favoured conservation and elaboration of genes for these basic functions. But there then must be an inherent, genetic risk of clonal escape. In these circumstances, the potency of natural selection might be a real liability.

The evolutionary emergence of multicellular organisms will have required an effective and stable resolution of this conflict between the individual cell and the conglomerate of cells in an individual – how to exploit the beneficial expansion of clones with specialized function within finite limits without giving free reign; how to stop cells resurrecting the historical imperative for selfish, self-perpetuation as individual clones. This evolutionary dilemma was much less acute for the emerging plant species that adopted different architectures from animals, with fixed or immobile cells with rigid cell walls. Here the opportunities for regression to a clonal individuality were intrinsically less. This provides a simple but plausible explanation of why plants can develop localized tumours but not cancers. But for the emerging metazoan animals with flexi-cells, the problem must have been acute. Not surprisingly therefore, there has been evolutionary pressure for the development of constraints to severely diminish this liability and risk.

These controls operate as a kind of social contract drawn up in the language of DNA and exercised by chemical signals emitted and received between different sorts of cells. Each type of cell in blood, brain, or elsewhere lives in its own sensory world, equivalent to the unique 'merkwelt' of each species (to plagiarize a term from animal behaviour). The received signals then collect-ively and reciprocally regulate what a cell is allowed to do, where and when – what song to sing. Cells can also sense what space is available to them, via adhesive contacts with neighbours and consequent mechanical tension. These essential controls serve to limit the clone size, territory, viability, and life span of individual cellular constituents, or clones. The imposition of these controls begins with the fertilized egg. Gradients of maternal chemicals provide unequal local environments within descendant cells that are then compelled to adopt alternative patterns of gene expression. This then initiates a cascade of sequential steps resulting in divergent cell specialization, a process referred to as differentiation and tissue morphogenesis. Orchestration of this develop-mental process of specialization in the embryo severely restricts but does not eliminate opportunities for clonal escape. It must be a balancing act as cell migration and clonal expansion have to be co-opted for beneficial purposes.

Solving this dilemma was a major turning point in evolution and the detailed solutions adapted were reflected in the elaboration of distinctively different animal architectures or 'bauplans'. Most of this process was complete by the pre-Cambrian period around 500 million years ago and most of what has happened since has been elaboration of the solutions that worked. Evolution-ary pressure would nevertheless, over time, result in the diversification and refinement of intercellular controls and clonal constraints, in so far as they enhance survival and reproductive fitness of the whole animal. More elaborate or stringent controls would have been adopted as animals lived longer, acquired more architecturally complex body forms with circulatory networks facilitating cell migration, and became more physiologically adaptable. But critically, from the perspective of cancer, continued resilience of function throughout life, after the embryonic body plan has been laid down, was 'dis-covered' to operate best if some cells were given a permit to remain only partially differentiated and to retain the potential for clonal expansion. This provides the mechanism by which longer-lived creatures such as ourselves can constantly, or on demand, replenish tissues that are subject to functional exhaustion or damage – a smart move in evolutionary terms but, as we shall see, a potentially cancerous legacy.

Overall, much of the evolutionary success of more complex animals has been attributed to the adoption of a design programme that may seem counter-intuitive: essential tissue functions are organized to reside on the edge of chaos, relatively stable but oscillating and primed for transient, regulated instability. The big bonus is flexibility, resilience, and maximum fitness. The down side of mismanagement is occasional one-way trips to the wrong side. Cancerous cell behaviour is one vivid example; blood clotting mechanisms, a belligerent immune system, and their pathological sideshows are others.

Death by design

Antagonizing potentially selfish clonal proliferation by the imposition of cell specialization or differentiation works. It is effective because the process terminates in cells that channel their energies into exercising specialist functions such as making digestive enzymes or contracting or transmitting nerve impulses, rather than making more copies of themselves. But there is another critical control that is perhaps less obvious and that is cell death. All cells of multicellular organisms have a genetically determined programme for committing suicide by a process called apoptosis, which involves self-digestion. Moreover, this intrinsic tendency will be acted out unless it is positively overruled by survival signals that can only be provided by other cells. This sounds an extraordinary and counter-intuitive arrangement, particularly for those of our cells that exercise vital functions, but it does make sense. The efficient regulation of our development as complex embryos and our continual physiological activity requires that cells die where and when appropriate. And, operationally, in the context of evolutionary trial and error, the giving or denying of a reprieve worked well.

Proper function of the embryo involves major structural modelling in which excess cells must be removed to ensure appropriate shape and function. Examples include the timed loss of the tadpole's tail and the removal of extra cells in the human foetal hand in order to convert a web-like structure to a hand with discrete fingers. After birth, the dynamic structure and turnover of the blood, skin, and epithelial surfaces (lung, gut, and hormonal glands) requires that rapid production and loss, by cell death and cell shedding, are balanced and can be regulated on demand. Additionally, apoptosis provides an efficient mechanism to remove cells that are damaged. Restricting cell numbers within sensible limits via cell suicide would a priori appear to limit the opportunity for any emerging cancer clone, particularly if cells with DNA that is damaged above a threshold level are compelled to commit suicide. It isn't difficult to see therefore why genes encoding mechanisms for promoting cell death were a useful and very early evolutionary adaptation, perhaps arising in colonial unicellular organisms. This functional logic explains why all our epithelial tissues and blood turn over so rapidly – here is the cellular venue for a perpetual confrontation with a toxic world and the likely focus for DNA damage.

But what if the built-in suicide programme develops a fault? Recent research has provided compelling evidence that aberrant regulation of cell death can have dire pathological consequences. Cells dying when they shouldn't is a major factor in neurodegenerative conditions, atherosclerosis, AIDS immune pathology, and autoimmune self-destruction of tissues. Cells not dying, when by all rights they should be sent packing, is a striking and crucial feature of cancerous clones. The emergence of a cancer clone reflects a progressive breakdown of the evolutionary contract maintaining the balance of clonal expansion and restraint in which cell death is a key regulator.

Design flaws and cancer risks

A number of important predictions for cancer follow from these basic design features of all multicellular animals including ourselves. First, that particular cells with extensive longevity, replicative potential, and migratory capacity should be most at risk of cancerous transformation. The cells concerned exist transiently in the developing embryo and foetus and, throughout life, in those tissues that are continually self-renewing, that proliferate on demand, or that can regenerate after injury (blood, skin, and the linings of lung, intestines, the endocrine glands, and liver). These specialized cells are called stem cells. Few in number and spawned in early development, these cells serve as the reservoir from which the clonal progeny can be generated by cell division when required to form or replenish these tissues. By the same token, the genes that normally exercise critical functions essential for proliferation and migration of these cells or the complementary restraining functions, would be expected to be the main molecular or DNA-based targets most at risk of mutation (or rather, when once mutated of being more likely than others to confer clonal advantage). This prediction is amply fulfilled as we shall see later.

A second prediction is that different tissues of the body will be maximally at risk at different times, in relation to peaks in their normal development and physiological activity, and this should be reflected in the age incidence of different types of cancer. In the developing embryo or foetus in the womb, the stem cells forming muscle, kidney, and parts of the nervous system such as the retina, and the sympathetic nervous system, will be at risk. But after birth, these cells cease to be vulnerable as their proliferative activity will largely have ceased; most, if not all of them, are dead or dormant. We don't need more of these cells. Hence muscle cancers (rhabdomyosarcomas) and eye tumours (retinoblastomas) are cancers of early childhood but exceedingly rare later in life.

Conversely, the equivalent stem cells in the blood, epithelial surfaces of skin, lung, and intestinal linings, and the endocrine, hormonal glands are active over decades in adults or throughout life and provide therefore a constant, if moving, target population of cells whose risk might be expected to be incremental with age. Hence the dominance of epithelial carcinomas in adult cancer. In this category, we see that women have a very rough deal indeed since the reproductive demands on the female body put at risk several vulnerable organs – breasts, ovaries, uterus, cervix, and vagina. Whereas for the male, it's the prostate gland, with its modest lubricating function, that appears most at risk in ageing men, along with relatively rare testicular cancer in younger men and very rare cancers of the penis. This sexual asymmetry has some dire consequences. If it wasn't for the fact that men have been out-smoking women for a long time, mortality from cancer would now be far higher for women than men – as it was in previous centuries.

In between these typical embryonic and adult cancers is bone cancer or osteosarcoma, where the maximum incidence and risk of disease is exactly when you might anticipate it – coincident with the adolescent spurt of long bone growth at 13–15 years. Whatever actually 'causes' cancer, its age-associated incidence is intimately linked to our genetically programmed development and function.

Trouble down in the genes

The evolutionary process itself is dependent upon genetic variation arising from mutation and, for sexual species, recombination or genetic exchanges which, like mutations, generate novel variation. But this now poses a real conundrum in the context of genetically regulated restraints against cancer: no changes in genes = no cancer; no changes in genes = no evolution = no us. The potential magnitude of this intrinsic and unavoidable risk looks at first sight very daunting.

Both germ cell repositories of chromosomal DNA destined for offspring and the rest of our diverse somatic cells have efficient mechanisms for replicating their DNA every time they divide in two. Duplication of DNA and the entire gene set requires faithful copying of the sequence of the four types of nucleotide bases (A, C, T, and G) that constitutes the genetic code. But very occasionally, a buffeting motion created by thermal energy prevents the correct base being inserted in the newly formed replicate. If and when an erroneous or mutated code is then translated by the cell, the result can be a protein with altered structure and function. This inherent and very ancient design limitation could have been a major problem but its impact is minimized since our cells are biochemically equipped to proofread, edit, and repair any errors in the DNA sequence that may arise spontaneously, or via mutagenic insult. But this process also lacks complete fidelity and mutations are inevitable, albeit at a low level and commensurate with potential added value for offspring beneficiaries of germ cell's DNA.

Roughly speaking, a small error or change in sequence will be inserted once in every one million copies of a gene that are made. This sounds minuscule and trivial until one grasps the fact that each day we make 10^{11} (that is, 100 000 million) blood cells by cell division and a similar number of cells in our small intestine. Copying each gene 10^{11} times means that many mistakes will inevitably be made and 10^{11} cells is an alarming number if only one mutant cell is required to generate a cancer. Consider also the number of genes at risk. We all have somewhere between 30 000 and 40 000 genes in each cell of our bodies. Many of these encode instructions for functions that are directly relevant to clonal expansion or restraint. So far, around 200 different genetic abnormalities have been implicated in human cancer; more will certainly emerge from a rapidly advancing molecular technology. So let's say 500 (or around 1 per cent) of our genes, when mutated, can acquire an altered function that contributes to cancer formation. Compound now the number of genes and cells at risk with the average lifespan of 75 years.

Now take on board, if you can bear it, the additional unsavoury facts. One, that microbial and plant toxins that can damage or cause mutations in cellular DNA are ubiquitous in nature and carry infectious or dietary greeting cards. Two, that our cellular metabolism generates molecular species of oxygen and nitrogen as byproducts that are also capable of genetic abuse if present in sufficient quantity or ineffectively neutralized. These deleterious chemical entities, including the colourfully named 'free radicals', are produced in some quantity by macrophages and other cells during the metabolic overdrive that occurs in inflammatory reactions. These being responses that are in a broader context beneficial. The real surprise is not that cancer is relatively common in an ageing population but that we don't all have multiple cancers at a very young age. Or that geriatric elephants and giant turtles aren't riddled with cancer. Or that we are here at all. Don't you agree?

Odds against

The explanation for this conundrum turns out to be straightforward enough and lies in the very demanding credentials required to qualify as a cancer gene and cancer cell. For a gene to contribute to cancer development:

1 it must mutate and be unrepaired or incorrectly repaired;

2 it must mutate in a fashion that results in an alteration in the function of the protein for which it codes;

3 that altered function must directly or indirectly provide a sustained reproductive advantage to the cell and its progeny;

4 the mutation should occur in a rare long-lived stem cell with intrinsic

proliferative potential. The same argument applies, in principle, to mutations in germ cells (sperm and egg precursors), that contribute to species diversification in evolution. Now, mutations in DNA are more or less random, blind, or non-adaptive with regard to their functional impact on cells or organisms. It follows then, with respect to these requirements, that the vast majority of mutations in the vast majority of cells are simply irrelevant. And finally, but crucially;

5 although only one mutant cell is ultimately sufficient to make a malignant cancer, one mutant gene is seldom, if ever, enough. Indeed, one mutant gene compelling proliferation may solicit penalty or protective responses of non-proliferative rest or apoptotic death. Several genetic abnormalities are usually required to act in concert, as a set, within the same cell. It is their co-operative or combinatorial function that engenders a malignant clone. More on this in a moment.

The odds are also stacked against stem cells incurring these mutations in the first place. Not surprisingly, evolution has provided these crucial, long-lived cells with some special protection. This comes in the form of stringent rules of engagement, some physical insulation, and then fail-safe devices. First of all, despite the fact that we produce such huge numbers of progeny each day from stem cells, these vital founder cells are numerically rare (less than 1 in 10 000 bone marrow cells is a blood stem cell) and they do not divide very much. How is this possible given the profligate daily output of new blood cells? After birth, stem cells spend much of their time in a state of non-dividing dormancy. This reduces risk substantially as non-replicating DNA is physically compacted within the chromosome structure and less vulnerable to damage. Different stem cells take turns at indulging in transient proliferation but the vast numbers of progeny produced each day derive not directly from excessive stem cell division but from some of the first descendants of stem cells. These immature cells are transitory, mortal cells but can undergo extensive cycles of replication before their daughter cells finally mature and stop dividing or die. A single mutation hit in one of these transitory cells, in whatever gene, is likely to be lost as the cells' descendants disappear. The restraining rule for an 'at risk' dividing stem cell is therefore a three-way choice of exit: stop dividing (and return to a dormant state); continue to divide but also start the process of running down by maturation (= terminal differentiation); or die.

Evolutionary adaptations also accommodate the hostile world in which our cells function. And the best tricks are the old ones. Our cells are the historical beneficiaries of two very ancient gambits that serve to diminish opportunities for mutagenic damage to DNA from either external or internal assault. The first line of protection lies in protein molecules that span cell surfaces and serve a kind of janitor function controlling influx and particularly efflux of foreign molecules. The recognition systems involved are relatively simple, based upon molecular attributes of shape and charge, but they ensure that potentially toxic molecules are pumped out of cells. Such a simple but effective trick for reducing the impact of genotoxic molecules makes much sense in an evolutionary context but was not appreciated until quite recently. As we shall see later, it has serious implications for attempts to cure cancer via genotoxic drugs. The other equally ancient cellular adaptation is a purging process, by which our cells can metabolize and neutralize potentially genotoxic molecules that have gained entry and similarly reduce or antioxidize potentially harmful byproducts of our endogenous oxidative metabolism. Cellular ablutions, in effect. Still, we all have some low-level unrepaired DNA injury arising through oxidative damage which suggests that our cellular capacity to neutralize or mop up can be satiated or bypassed.

These are general tactics for ensuring cell survival. Stem cells need and receive some additional help. The physical location of stem cells in intestinal epithelia, for example (at the very base of small crypts away from the exposed surfaces or lumens) reduces their exposure to potentially damaging toxins and mutagenic substances as well as restraining their territory. And then if these cells do incur DNA damage, they have an efficient and altruistic fail-safe device – they activate a suicidal cell death programme. Smart eh? The level of damage that initiates quick death seems to vary between different tissues as judged by their differential sensitivity to radiation. Some stem cells, for example in the small intestine (where turnover of cells is very rapid and sustained), in the lymphocyte development pathway (bone marrow and thymus), and our primitive germ cells (the sperm and egg precursors), are exquisitely sensitive to a very small number of breaks in DNA and die when damaged. This has the hallmark of very prudent planning with respect to cancer risk. The germ cells and primitive lymphocytes are the only stem cells in the body that generate offspring that themselves have stem cell-like properties of longevity and proliferative potential. They do need to be kept on a tight leash. Even so, these cells can develop into cancers – but not nearly as often as their florid and persistent activity might imply.

Stem cells are therefore under constant surveillance and protection. But their normal physiological function, over decades in humans, requires remarkable resilience and adaptability. They can, under some circumstances, be pushed to the limit – and then, over the edge.

Gambling with sex

One further evolutionary gambit was required to restrain the deleterious effect of mutations that might unleash a genetic prescription for clonal escape. You don't want mutations like this in your germ line to pass on to descendants. It paid therefore to organize cell specification in early embryos so that the cell lineage responsible for transporting DNA to the next generation was hived off and sequestered in a small number of specialized (germ) cells – a process that in humans takes place around six weeks after conception. But then we have the dilemma: it is in these very cells that all the potential for future beneficial variation and evolution resides. Once again, a trade-off or balancing act had to be executed as an early evolutionary adaptation of multicellular organisms. Preventing excessive mutant load by cell death imposition was one trick. But the really clever ploy was sex.

In species or clones that reproduce asexually, the load of mutations in progeny, including some that can be deleterious, can only move in one direction – upwards. This is referred to by evolutionary biologists as Muller's Ratchet after the geneticist Hermann Muller. In contrast, for a sexual reproducing species there is a shuffling within the parental gene sets. The individual is reconstructed anew and offspring can be generated that lack a mutation that was present in one of the parental germ lines. Sexual reproduction, it is argued, increased fitness of (some) offspring by purging mutations. At the same time, this process could introduce further genetic variation by exchanges of DNA between the genomes (or by more conventional mutation). The end result of these evolutionary gambits is, however, still a trade-off: mutations are still generated, and indeed facilitated, but distributed differentially in offspring. The luck of the draw then operates with, in stark Darwinian terms, survival of the fittest.

Overall the gamble must have paid given the prevalence of sexual species on our planet. But it does mean that some cancer-causing mutations can arise during specification of the germ line and be passed on to some, but not all, offspring. You might expect such mutations to be effectively lost in our predecessors if they resulted in death of the offspring. Unfortunately, for us, it's not so simple. First, because of the evolutionary requirements of the cancer clone itself, emergence of a life-threatening cancer, initiated by an inherited mutant gene, can be delayed until after the silent mutant gene has been passed on again to the next generation of offspring. Second, new potentially cancerous mutations will be acquired in the germ line all the time at some frequency. The consequence is that we inherit a burden of cancer contributing directly to perhaps 5 to 10 per cent of all cancers combined. Evolution has no malign intent; it's just the way it works, blindfolded to consequences.

A reprise

Cancerous cell behaviour is an inherent legacy of our evolutionary and developmental history. Certain types of cells normally exercise this pattern of behaviour, albeit subject to stringent social constraints of time and space. Our complex tissue architecture and resilience or adaptability of function is in fact contingent upon these 'dangerous' properties. The social contract between cells that minimizes risk of clonal escape is underpinned, in common with all other biological rules of engagement, by genetic legislation encoded in DNA or genes. But the code is not sacrosanct. It can be damaged or corrupted despite the existence of ancient and efficacious mechanisms for editing, maintenance, and repair of DNA and for cellular cleansing. Cancer then becomes a statistical inevitability in nature – a matter of chance and necessity, to quote Jacques Monod's memorable phrase applied to evolution. In one sense the real surprise is that cancer hasn't always been much more common.

This perspective begs an obvious question that moves us closer to some practical realities: if cancer is an accident of our evolutionary heritage (a design fault), what parameters influence the risk of this actually happening in your or my lifetime? And what can we do about it? But before we can address these crucial questions, we need to look at how cancer cells actually succeed in escaping. This will be a somewhat mechanical explanation as revealed by the extraordinary advances in molecular biology of the past 25 years. The dynamic picture it allows us to construct resets the frame for considering the grander questions of causes and control.

CHAPTER 8

HOW CANCER CELLS PLAY THE WINNING GAME

Evolutionary bottlenecks

To generate a fully-fledged or dominant cancer clone, a cell has to subvert multiple rules of engagement and negotiate major evolutionary bottle- necks. For most types of cancer, this is only possible by the accumula- tion of a set of mutations in genes exercising different, but complementary or interlocking, functions. Because of the statistical rarity of DNA damage creating one of these mutations and because accrual of a set of mutations is only possible by sequential addition, the process can only operate in single cells, or clonally and over an extended period of time. This makes the whole process probabilistic and pervaded by chance (Fig. 8.1).

Paradoxically perhaps, the multiple and stringent restraints on clonal expansion that have been assembled by evolutionary selection themselves pro- vide the potent microenvironmental pressures begetting natural selection of individual mutant cells; that is, those that can evade controls or outpace neigh- bours. Cancer cells can adopt manoeuvres that reduce dependency upon, or subjugation to, their local environments or they can alter their local environ- ments to provide a more fertile soil for expansion. These are in fact natural and physiologically useful adaptive responses in their proper context and time frame. The trouble comes from the generation and selection of mutants that are impervious to context.

The first bottleneck venue for confrontation and selection is within the cancer cell itself. The emergence of a dominant clone from a stem cell pool obviously requires a reproductive advantage. But a mutation that encourages a cell to persist in making more of itself by division is not enough. This is because of the imposition of preprogrammed internal restraints that are signalled in response to cell proliferation. Unless the normally integrated processes of proliferation and restraint are effectively uncoupled, reproductive advantage itself will be minimal or unsustained; increased cell proliferation driven by a mutant gene will usually prompt or lead to exhaustion, differentiation, and slumber in a non-dividing quiescent state or cell death. Prospects for clonal emancipation are then poor, particularly if the cell is dead. The most that can be achieved in this situation is a resetting of the dynamic equilibrium, both increased cell division followed downstream by a compensatory increase in cell death. The result then is a modest size tumour with essentially normal cellular architecture and function. Such a tumour, for example a polyp, may appear dormant but the lack of continued growth reflects a stand-off between the opposing forces of proliferation and cell death. Nevertheless, such a clonal tumour has taken one first step towards clonal escape and malignancy.[4]

For a clone to dominate, production must outpace loss, and the big trick is to co-opt complementary mutations that allow proliferation to proceed without imposition of penalties. In principle therefore, many mutations involved in cancer are of two basic types: those that directly provoke reproductive activity of cells, often in a constitutive or unrelenting manner (the stuck accelerator pedal metaphor), and those resulting in loss of some important penalty imposition or restraining functions (the faulty brake metaphor).[5] The latter can include defects in cell multiplication inhibitors, a failure of differentiation induction, and a loss of access to senescence or suicidal cell death pathways. Restraining adhesive contacts with neighbouring cells may also be reduced. There is then a strong selective pressure in cancer in favour of single cells that acquire a complementary set of mutations that collectively provide for sustained proliferation plus diminished restraint. Stringent, or even partial, blocking of growth arrest, differentiation, and cell death pathways in a constitutively dividing clone will have more selective advantage than removing any one of these restraining influences alone. Loss of these exit routes will trap more of the clone in the proliferating stem cell compartment. Clonal proliferation can now be sustained without the penalty of compulsory retirement or death. The Red Queen's dilemma then applies:

> Now, here, you see, it takes all the running you can do, to keep in the same place.
> (The Red Queen to Alice in *Through the Looking Glass* by Lewis Carroll)[6]

Trapping more dividing cells at the top, stem cell, end of the lineage hierarchy has two other crucial consequences. First, these dividing cells are not normally programmed to follow the same rules of residential engagement as their mature descendants. They are primed to be more mobile and independent. As expanding clones they reveal their juvenile aspirations by failing to construct a normal functional architecture. To a pathologist looking down a microscope, the tumour or 'carcinoma *in situ*' will have many dividing immature-looking cells and will have an irregular shape disrupting normal architecture and impinging on surrounding tissue. Pathologists have trad-

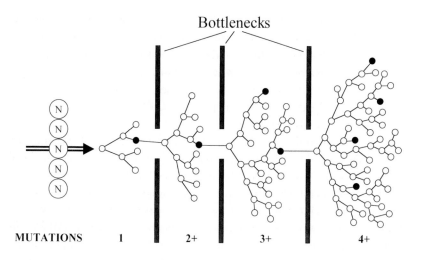

Figure 8.1 Clonal evolution of a cancer. A model of the sequential acquisition of mutations (1–4+) in a clone of cancer cells as it evolves, left to right, through bottlenecks providing selective pressure. Each black cell represents a new mutation. N = normal stem cell.

itionally interpreted this disorganized or poorly differentiated state in a cancerous tissue as a sign of dedifferentiation, or going backwards. But pathological snapshots disguise dynamics. A second and crucial consequence of running in the same place is that more stem cells are dividing, providing more opportunity for further mutation and clonal evolution.

The selective pressure that begets the natural selection of cancer cells comes at them from all sides, and from within. First, within the proliferating cancer clone itself, nature's contingency plan to impose exit rules of cell slumber or suicide provides the context in which any mutant that can find a way to turn a blind eye to these penalty clauses will gain an instant advantage over its more mortal neighbours. As any founder clone expands, space and nutrients may well become limited providing further opportunity and selective pressure for the emergence of any cell that adopts mutant tricks to outpace its normal and cancerous siblings. This it can do, for example, by becoming more sensitive to lower levels of critical growth factors, by becoming insensitive to negative growth regulators, by synthesizing its own growth factors, or by inducing the surrounding tissue cells to produce more supportive growth factors – by altering its environment. By cheating, in other words.

A complementary set of mutations is then a formula for sustained reproductive advantage – a bottleneck negotiated. But not a complete prescription. Simply staying put and growing bigger and bigger is not necessarily an effective or winning strategy for a cancer clone, as also applies for individual animals, termite mounds, or our social institutions. Cancer cells in an expanding tumour may be dysregulated and antisocial but they are still subject to some rather unavoidable laws of physics and chemistry. They need oxygen and space. The faulty accelerator and brake may propel our vehicle relentlessly forward but we still need a fuel supply and some space on the road. The diffusion properties of oxygen and nutrients in physiological fluids are such that any cell, aberrant or not, finds it difficult to survive and multiply if more than a milli-metre or so away from the supply source (blood capillaries). This then imposes a significant evolutionary bottleneck on a cancer clone's expansionist tendency to sustain growth beyond a few cubic millimetres. The formation of new blood capillary function must be solicited – a process called *angiogenesis* (see Fig. 8.2). This bloody process is prompted by both oxygen-deficient or anoxic con-ditions suffocating tumours and by the production by cancer cells of growth factors that induce vascular cell proliferation. This is corruption, in the clonal cause, of a normally innocent or physiological process that has evolved to facilitate inflammation and wound healing as well as tissue assembly in the embryo and function of the cycling ovary and placenta in mammals.

There is another striking paradox in this impoverished microenvironment and anoxic graveyard of struggling tumours. Deficiency of blood supply leads

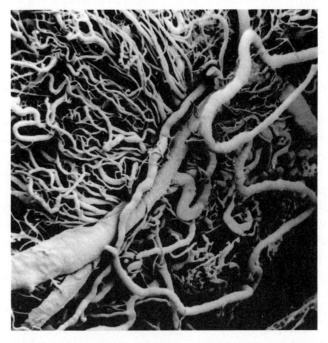

Figure 8.2 Bloody sustenance. Stereoscan electron microscopic image of vascular blood vessels surrounding and nourishing a tumour.

to oxygen deprivation and cell death which must apply a brake on clonal expansion. But at the same time as invoking vascular rescue, these conditions may provide selective pressure favouring expansion of any pre-existing mutant that can survive this kind of stress. Mutants in the *p53* gene, a major player in cancer clone evolution that we'll hear about later, may emerge as dominant subclones via this mechanism. There is also some evidence that anoxic conditions trigger breakage of DNA and, for surviving cells, bequeath a heritage of increased genetic diversity and fitness for selection. Once new blood capillary formation clicks in with oxygen and nutrient-sufficient conditions in their wake, tumours, or a new mutant subclone thereof, expand, sometimes to a remarkable size. But in most locations they will still eventually find themselves in a physical strait-jacket.

Rights of passage

Even if physiological constraints on expansion have been subverted – the brakes off, the red light ignored – there are still roadblocks in the way of cancer clones. Our tissues are structured into physical compartments rather than open plan. Fibrous proteins and matrices define boundaries and barriers within which cells are normally parked, with limited space for manoeuvre – the equivalent for an overpopulating and localized species of animal of a surrounding mountain range, or, for those on a small island, the surrounding sea. Another big bottleneck. The trick is of course to emigrate. And fortunately (or unfortunately, depending how you look at it) the escape routes and inter-tissue highways are already in place, for sound evolutionary and physiological reasons, and therefore available for exploitation. Angiogenesis undoubtedly facilitates this process both by enhancing numbers of would-be migrants and by providing direct exit routes or increased physical pressure in the tumour that encourages transit of cells into draining lymphatics.

But what's still needed for negotiating this next evolutionary bottleneck for a cancer cell is an exit passport, a survival strategy for swimming in a turbulent stream, and an entry visa for a new location. Genes encoding these requirements are there also; what the cancer cell has to do as its next trick is indulge in a bit of forgery or smuggling. Cell migrants would normally be denied passports but by expressing the appropriate migrant phenotype, cells can reduce adhesive neighbourhood contacts, enzymatically degrade physical barriers, enter the bloodstream or lymphatic circulation, infiltrate other tissues, and set up camp. Proliferating stem cells may normally express the migratory, non-adherent and barrier-breaching instincts that are required for emigration but it is likely that further mutations facilitate this process. In particular, given the partly foreign territory that has to be crossed, cells that have already abrogated the cell death response to stressful signals will be at a decided advantage. But even when armed with these credentials, it is rather like a desperate migrant crossing the China Sea in a fragile vessel; very few will make it. But given the number that try and the time available, inevitably a few may succeed.

Dissemination of a cancer clone, or metastasis, is not an all or nothing event but happens in stages or as a cascade. The initial migration of a carcinoma will often be to local lymph nodes serving as a transit camp for expansion and then subsequent dissemination. Liver, lung, and bone then become preferred sites of secondary residence with other tissues as tertiary sites. There is clearly some selectivity in the patterns of colonization of tissues. This appears to be in part explained by the anatomical constraints and traffic flow rules of the lymphatics and vasculature within which escapees will follow the line of least resistance. Cancer cells may flow within the bloodstream as small aggregates or emboli of cells and become arrested in the first major capillary bed they encounter. They may also actively migrate to tissues that release chemo-attractant molecules into the blood. Successfully establishing a base for further incursions and expansion within a new tissue is more demanding. Few migrating cancer cells are truly autonomous in their ecological requirements. Success, by clonal expansion, is more likely in a similar environment or ecosystem to that from which it came – one part of the bladder to the other, skin to skin. If this were a species of animal expanding its territory, we would refer to it as habitat tracking. Failing the availability of an identical environment, cancer cells will be more likely to survive and expand in sites that have both the space and are nutrient-rich. Hence our bones, lung, and liver provide convenient and accessible niches for expansion of melanomas, breast and prostate cancer clones (see Fig. 8.3).

But these environments are still foreign. Clonal expansion may occur inefficiently and more slowly; selfish ploys may be advantageous. These can include co-opting local signals for growth normally reserved for specialized residents and provoking damage and repair processes. For example, in bony metastases, infiltrating cancer cells solicit activation of bone resorption and remodelling processes releasing growth factors predestined for repair but usurped by the colonizer. An alternative tactic is to become more self-sufficient by making self-stimulating molecules, functionally replacing those usually pro-vided by other local cells as part of normal social dialogue. As in all colonialist excursions, there is a dialogue of some sort between the invader and the invaded but, in the short term at least, natural selection will favour the more manipulative intruder who can alter local conditions in its favour.

With all the tricks in the book to exercise their imperialistic tendencies, disseminated cancer clones still require oxygen. New immigrant clones are often perivascular in distribution, hovering around their nutrient- and oxygen-

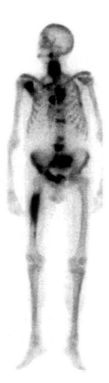

Figure 8.3 Cancer clone metastasis: a territorial hijack. Gamma camera image of skeletal metastasis of prostate cancer (the black areas) using a metabolic tracer. This type of imaging is used clinically for disease stage and selection of therapy.

rich entry point. But those clones will usually not continue to expand unless they can again recruit new blood vessel formation or perchance find themselves in naturally vascularized beds of tissue. So, in the absence of angiogenesis, these 'micrometastases' tend to remain micro and effectively dormant, still proliferating at source but with minimal expansion as cell death under anoxic conditions matches cell gain by proliferation. Curiously, angiogenic activity in the primary tumour can, via blood-borne chemical mediators, competitively suppress blood vessels in the new locales. This perhaps explains the long-standing, paradoxical finding that surgical extirpation of the primary tumour can sometimes accelerate development of distant, metastatic disease.

Passing through the emigration bottleneck is *the* critical evolutionary event in cancer – both for the clone and the patient. The dominant clone, or rather subclone, now exercises its expansionist tendency and the consequence is a territorial hijack of essential organs, a compromise of normal functions, and associated morbidity. To have reached this stage of evolution via natural selection the cancer clone will have expanded, mutated, and diversified sufficiently to have become robust and resilient. This sets them up, rather serendipitously, to negotiate *the* major bottleneck in a now unnatural history – intervention by the oncologist. Hence the unfortunate but inevitable failure of most therapeutic interventions in patients with advanced or metastatic cancer. We'll see how exactly cancer cells escape the therapeutic axe later in this book (Part Four). It's a salutary and sorry tale but one that is entirely consistent with the evolutionary paradigm. At the same time, new opportunities arise from our appreciation of the processes involved. For example, the apparently invariant requirement of even widely disseminated cancer clones for sustenance from newly formed blood vessels provides one of the most promising new lines of therapeutic intervention. It's not all gloomy news.

There is one other important source of selective pressure that can promote the evolutionary selection or emergence of cancer clones. This derives from toxic environmental insults that form part of the aetiological pathway for cancer. Many of the environmental substances or agents that are implicated in the causation of cancer are poisonous or toxic; some are mutagenic *and* toxic. Examples would be damage to the bone marrow by chemicals such as benzene and some viral infections, a number of liver-damaging chemicals as well as hepatitis B virus, chemicals in cigarette tar that are toxic to the lung linings, and gastritis caused by high-salt diets or bacterial infection. There is both experimental and clinical evidence that the development of cancer in these organs may be preceded by an aplasia or loss of cells followed by regeneration and repair. Under these circumstances there will be selective pressure favouring any mutant cells that are resistant to toxic stress or that can outpace others in the regenerative race to reoccupy the space vacated by toxic clearance. Evolutionary biologists recognize that there is nothing like a bit of environmental decimation for encouraging the phoenix-like emergence of new and diversified species. Especially weed species.

Our own defensive and reparative processes can be subverted into this pathway of cancer pathogenesis to inadvertently provide a mutational boost to the risk of a cancerous clone emerging during periods of cell recovery. Inflammatory reactions in which our macrophages, neutrophils, and other white blood cells invade infected or damaged tissue are a defence system that evolved from parallel, albeit simpler, defence systems in invertebrates. The potency of these cells in executing their clean-up activities is associated with high-energy turnover and production of reactive oxygen species as byproducts. As a transient blip, these can be tolerated but they are potentially damaging to DNA. It has been known for some time that persistent inflammatory lesions are a risk factor for some cancers. It's now clear how this link operates: a high proportion of patients with pancreatitis, ulcerative colitis, or gastritis that is chronic or of several years' standing have mutational changes in the epithelial regions subjected to this stand-off between damage and repair. Ironically, collateral damage is caused by a natural biological process adapted for its beneficial attributes.

It therefore appears that several kinds of toxic insults both create tissue microenvironmental conditions for competitive survival and clonal recovery *and* directly or indirectly induce the mutations that give the competitive edge. Now that's what I call dangerous. And guess what else commonly has these undesirable double attributes. It's cancer therapy.

And for my final trick: how about immortality?

So here we are with a set of rules of the game for the 'natural' selection of cancer cells. But there is yet one more twist in the tail. This concerns the desirable attribute shared by simple creatures that clonally propagate, and by angels – immortality. It turns out that most, if not all, human cells have a built-in 'clock' that counts cell divisions and sets an upper limit. The clock hands correspond to the end of chromosomes that erode slightly with every division. When their time is up, cells senesce, are compelled to sleep or die, which is not a very profitable career for a cancer cell. So there will obviously be very considerable selective pressure for any cancer cell that can stop the clock ticking. This it can do by activating an enzyme that rejuvenates chromosome ends following each cell division. Whether this is a mutational step isn't yet clear since some of our stem cells normally express this 'immortality' enzyme, called telomerase, but it is a critical property acquired by all malignant clones. The prize is immortality. More on this a little later on.

Collecting a full house

We still don't have a complete catalogue of genes, that as mutants or when lost or deleted, can contribute to cancer clone evolution. It is also unclear exactly how many mutations make a full set and prescription for unbridled clonal dominance or full malignancy. Generally speaking, the more advanced a cancer is in terms of its histopathological appearance or dissemination, the greater will be the number of detectable abnormalities or mutations within the dominant clone. But what, in this particular poker game, constitutes a full house?

To some extent you can only see what you look for in this situation, by fishing with very selective baits. It is therefore inevitable that the number of genetic abnormalities in a cancer cell and the diversity of such mutations within a clone is underestimated. This situation is however in the process of changing in the wake of technological advances. The human genome project, the development of micro-arrays of thousands of gene sequences, chromosome gene painting methods, and the National Cancer Institute's ambitious cancer genome anatomy project are some of the current advances that will revolutionize the way that human genes are interrogated. Complete genetic profiles of cancer cells should soon be achievable. At the moment we don't know the number of mutations that constitute a full house. The number could vary depending upon the cell type involved and the particular mutant cards that are dealt. At present, most cancer biologists are guessing that the number for most adult epithelial cancers once invasive or metastatic (that is, at the point of no return) is somewhere between 5 and 10. To be dealt a set of this size and special content, one card at a time, obviously takes time – a long time.

The requirement for a set or full house of genetic events or mutations, each of which is extremely rare or unlikely, helps explain why the statistical odds are stacked heavily against a dominant cancer clone emerging, why it usually takes a long time, and involves a clone derived from a single cell – why cancer is, in effect, a chronic disease. In fact a cursory consideration of mutation rates and simple calculations might suggest it should be impossible. And it would be if all mutations had to occur, by chance, simultaneously. But it doesn't work like that. To begin with, if the first mutation generates a clone of, say, 10 million cells, it only requires one out of these ten million to incur a second hit or 'appropriate' mutation to generate the next quasi-species or subclone which then becomes the expanded venue for hit number 3. And so on for hits 4 and 5 up to the full house for malignancy in a single cell.[7] The process therefore involves clonal succession and enormous redundancy or cell loss. Secondly, there will also be selective pressure in cancer clone evolution favouring an altogether different class of mutation – in housekeeping (or caretaker) genes. These maintain the integrity of chromosomes and DNA, that is, damage detection, repair, and stability, chromosome segregation at cell division (mitosis), and global regulation of gene expression. As mutants, these deleted or misdirected genes can confer widespread genomic instability, increasing the risk and rate of mutation by a hundred fold – a kind of evolutionary accelerator. One of the key genes here, with a star billing in cancer genetics, is called *p53* (see box).

For whom the bell tolls: the p53 gong

There is only one gene of the many involved in cancer that I am going to tell you anything at all about. It has a name like a bus – *p53* – which belies its extraordinary role in the life and death of cells. And in cancer.

Cells of all vertebrate species have a gene that encodes a protein called p53 (p for protein, 53 for 53K daltons molecular weight). The protein was discovered serendipitously by its interaction with a virus that caused tumours in animals. p53 protein is normally synthesized and degraded very rapidly by cells. However, when cells are damaged or stressed by any one of many different mechanisms, p53 is stabilized and is able to exercise its function as an alarm system. It then initiates different processes dependent upon cell type and level of insult. The underlying and prudent rule is that when cells are stressed and the integrity of DNA is seriously challenged, then proliferating cells must either:

1 pause and repair the damage, or

2 stop proliferating and enter a prolonged resting or quiescent state, or

3 leave the stage permanently – that is, drop dead.

A malfunction in the p53 alarm is very bad news. Mice without a functional *p53* gene (engineered by gene knockout technology) can suffer very high rates of congenital malformation following genotoxic stress. This suggests a plausible explanation for the evolutionary adaptive function of *p53*: that it could monitor cellular stress and DNA damage, via for example microbial or plant toxins, and signal either rescue via DNA repair or, if cell death is excessive, loss of the embryo. Better dead than red hot with mutations. A genotoxic insult, by ionizing radiation, to mouse embryos that are p53 deficient generates not only a plethora of different congenital mutants but a high rate of cancers, particularly leukaemias. An evolutionary bonus of stress and damage surveillance by p53 is therefore that it diminishes prospects for cancer clone emancipation via genotoxic damage. But then this credit rating means that abrogation of this protective function is the focus of considerable selective pressure in human cancer cell evolution. We see this in operation in different guises. Some individuals inherit a mutant variety of one copy of their pair of parental *p53* genes. Such individuals have the Li-Fraumeni syndrome which includes an increased risk of several forms of cancer (breast carcinomas, sarcomas, and leukaemias) relatively early in life. Some 50 per cent of non-familial, that is common, cancers have abnormalities of one or both copies of the *p53* gene (mutated or deleted) in the cancer cell clone. *p53* has the accolade of being the most commonly altered gene in human cancer. And it's not difficult to see how natural selection can bring this eminence about.

Absence of p53 function can:

1 allow cells to survive the otherwise deleterious impact of other mutations that compel persistent proliferation, that is, p53 loss complements other mutations;

2 allow cells to survive anoxic conditions, for example, in poorly vascularized tumours;

3 allow some cancer-causing viruses to replicate, for example, papilloma virus 16 in cervical cancer;

4 allow cells to survive and continue to divide in the presence of DNA damage, for example, cells in sunburnt skin.

The presence of a genetic abnormality in the *p53* gene in a cancer biopsy is also a harbinger of poor clinical outcome of systemic chemotherapy or radiotherapy, probably because cells are then blind to DNA damage and fail to operate the fail-safe device of cell death.

Not for nought has p53 been called the guardian of our genome. Without it, cancer cells are on a roll and we are in big trouble.

This acceleration process happens too in normal microbial evolution. It can pay bacteria to release restraints on mutation frequency in a rapidly changing or hostile environment. It's called the SOS response. Some cancer biologists have argued that without the agency of a mutation accelerator, or a 'mutator' phenotype, then the evolution of a cancer clone via the accumulation of several independent mutations is a mathematical impossibility. A more sophisticated mathematical appraisal suggests that genetic instability is not an absolute requirement for generating mutational diversity within clones acquiring cancerous credentials or the accumulation of a full set of mutations in cancer clones – given enough time for clonal expansion and natural selection within these clones.[8] Still, widespread genomic instability is a striking feature of some types of cancer, particularly those of the gastro-intestinal tract. There is evidence that although the consequence of this feature, once acquired, may be plasticity for further advantageous change, its initial Darwinian selection may be an outcome of exposure to toxic chemicals in the gut. These both damage DNA *and* provide the selective pressure for mutants that bypass DNA repair in favour of cell survival.

Playing to win by sheer force of numbers is a common blitzkrieg policy employed by unicellular organisms and parasites and, to some extent, by most animal species (mammals and birds being the exceptions) that produce large numbers of offspring with the anticipation that a few will survive whatever. But the gambit in cancer is not just big numbers. One formula for success in cancer clones is simply this: lots of cells × lots of inheritable diversity. Ecological stress, competition, and natural selection will then tease out the rare clone and its progeny that can emerge as fully fledged cancers, carrying the full house of mutant cards that have given it the adaptive edge.

But, as always in biology, there is something that appears not to fit, another conundrum to resolve. If the probability of a full hand of mutant cards being dealt to a single cell is very low, involves complex clonal population dynamics, and generally takes decades, how is it possible that young infants and children get cancer at all? In a minority of cases, the process is kick-started by the inheritance of a mutant gene – but this doesn't usually happen. Neither is there evidence of early imposition of rampant genetic instability. So here's another explanation to ponder. Children seldom develop adult-type cancers of the epithelial surfaces in gut, lung, and skin, and endocrine tissues. Their cancers tend to arise, albeit at low frequencies, in cells and tissues that are very active in early development (the central nervous system, muscle, kidneys, and blood).

For children diagnosed at age around three with leukaemia, for example, mutations characteristic of the leukaemic clone are already there and detectable at birth. Moreover, the target cells involved are not only actively proliferating in early life but are required to be actively mobile and to some extent invasive (in order for our body form to take proper function and shape). Their local microenvironments are not only permissive for these activities but actively encourage them. Up to a point. This suggests the following possibility: that many cancers of early childhood require fewer (say only two) genetic events to provide lift-off to effective dissemination and clonal dominance. In particular, these cells might not be subject to the selective conditions favouring survival mutants in static tumours with anoxia. And as mobile cells, they may not have to evade the strict territorial confines or rules of residence imposed upon stem cells in the mature and structured epithelial tissues of adults.

Paediatric cancers may have therefore a rather different evolutionary history and promote diagnostic symptoms relatively early in their clonal trajectory. If this view is correct, as I believe it likely to be, then it not only explains how childhood cancers can develop in such a short time frame but also has important implications for the likelihood of therapy being curative, as we will see later.

Networking

Proliferation and the restraining functions of quiescence, differentiation or death are alternative and pliable responses of cells. Decisions to indulge in these activities are regulated by a very complex, genetically encoded network of signals that cascade within the cell to its central control at the level of DNA in the nucleus.[9]

Consider for example the simple relay depicted in Fig. 8.4, in which a series of chemical signals interpret and convert a stimulus (1) coming from outside the cell into a cell proliferation or Go response. For the initial signal (1) to be transmitted to its final destination in the cell nucleus requires a cascade of energy transfers via checkpoints, similar in some respects to relays and switches in an electric circuit. Each step involves protein–protein interaction or protein complexes, often with catalytic or enzyme function. The more appropriate metaphor for the whole ensemble is that of a complex protein *machine* with moving and interactive parts. And the analogy isn't as superficial as you might suppose. The three-dimensional interaction between different proteins at the 'nodal' decision points can be visualized via the power of X-ray diffraction analysis of their structures after converting the proteins into crystals. Some regions of the molecules have scaffold functions, others are clefts, crevices or bulges that serve for docking. Docking is followed by shape changes in one or more partners and further changes in molecular affiliations. These may influence the physical accessibility of the region(s) (i.e. open or closed) involved in a downstream interaction in the signal pathway or may reroute the molecule within the cell.

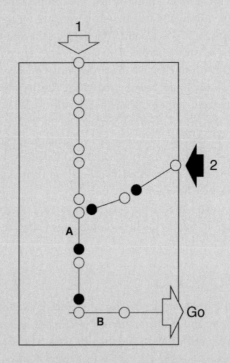

Fig. 8.4 Each step in the signalling relay involves a molecule that when activated by association with one or more partners (○) either activates (○—○) or inhibits (○—●) the next molecule in line, again by physical union. A critical point, as visualized in our simple model, is when component A is triggered: it then inhibits an inhibitor: the effect is that the signal B that releases *Go* is now released from repression. The final step in the 'get ready to *Go*' signal sequence is usually an interaction between protein complexes and the genetic machinery itself, DNA.

We cannot yet watch this process happening in real time but the mechanism appears to be, well, mechanics. In one sense, these molecular assemblies are in fact considerably more complex than man-made machines or circuits as they are continuously assembled and disassembled at the signal relay points. Indeed, it is the variable dynamics of this process that by and large determine activity in the signal circuit and resultant cell behaviour.

Such a relay will be networked, in the cell, with other signals controlling additional functions that can antagonize increased cell reproduction (via signal 2 in Fig. 8.4), including those that 'sense' precocious proliferation and divert otherwise proliferating cells down alternative response pathways of dormancy, cell death or differentiation. If we could visualize the complete patterns of the network in individual cells, we would see many zones and relays shared by very different types of cells. These might, for example, be signal components involved in cell proliferation or cell death. Their widespread usage reflects the conservation of evolutionarily ancient and efficacious rules underpinning common cellular functions. Other relays and components would appear more unique or idiosyncratic. These subserve specialized functions in particular cell types, for example, signals linked to cell–cell liaisons or differentiation.

This composite network within each cell type is not an isolated or independent entity. It is linked, via cell surface molecules that have receptor or decoding function, with signals from other cells within the micro-environments of each tissue. These unique habitats in turn are networked with whole body signal relays, hormones in the blood for example, that regulate and harmonize cellular and tissue function. And then the whole, Russian doll-like edifice is subject to multiple signals from outside the body. From within this cacophony of chemical chatter, signals can be selectively received and transduced as coded cues. When these are then integrated, the result is (usually) prudent cell behaviour. Complex, maybe, but how else could cells work if they are to be resilient and adaptive? But then this type of hierarchical structure delineates the multi-dimensional space or pitch on which oscillations and disturbances are acted out and where opportunities for cancerous proclivities can emerge.

The proper governance of our cells is dependent upon the integrity of these complex genetic circuits. Each individual protein component in this network is encoded by its own gene, any one of which, when mutated, may impact critically on the signal relay by altering molecular affiliations or deleting a link in the chain of command. Networking will usually ensure that fail-safe devices are triggered to minimize the impact of any individual fault or lesion. But when multiple components in these interlocked networks are corrupted by mutation within a single cell and its descendent progeny, then there is real trouble afoot. It is the progressive corrosion of this regulatory network that empowers clonal emancipation. The cells may still 'read' individual signals correctly but the signal–response pathways will now be uncoupled with respect to the functional logic of the whole system, i.e. its physiological context or rationale.

This picture helps to explain why so many genes can, in total, contribute as mutants to cancer development, why clonal advantage is maximized by mutations operating in concert within a single cell and why dysregulation of signals can convert a normally innocent or adaptive cellular function into one empowering clonal escape and dominance.

CHAPTER 9

ST PEREGRINE'S PROGRESS

Linear acceleration?

Cancer biologists often pictorialize cancer development as a simple linear sequence of mutational steps coupled with progressive selection of increasingly dominant subclones. This provides a time-ordered parallel with the progression of disease that the pathologist can recognize and grade in a biopsy section as disruption of tissue architecture and spread of disease. It also fits with an astute prediction by mathematically minded epidemiologists, Armitage and Doll, in the 1950s, that the exponential increase with age in most incidence of common forms of cancer was most probably a function of the time needed to accumulate a set of mutations in the subclone that eventually dominates at diagnosis.

Studies on the molecular pathogenesis of colon cancer by Bert Vogelstein and his colleagues at Johns Hopkins University Medical School have been particularly informative in this regard, and the lessons learnt probably apply to most adult cancer types. By comparing the molecular genetic profiles of colon cancer cells at sequential stages in their histopathological evolution from adenomas through to invasive carcinomas (in biopsies from different patients), it was possible to align, in parallel, the accumulative occurrence of genetic alterations. The latter then appears as a preferential, though not invariant, sequence of genetic mishaps. Other studies on normal as well as cancerous colon and rectum epithelium have suggested that small tumours or mini-adenomas are preceded by more numerous polyps that in turn are the descendants of dysplastic foci which in their turn are generated from within a more expansive population of aberrant, thickened intestinal crypts. Most of these very early lesions bear mutations in the *RAS* gene in the precise coding position that is observed in advanced cancers, as in that of the King of Naples. These patterns, revealed by endoscopy, biopsy, and histopathology and mutation screening, therefore provide a series of snapshots of a plausible evolutionary trajectory for colo-rectal cancers (see Fig. 9.1).

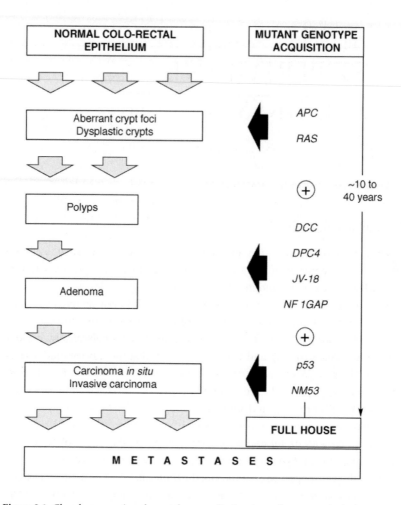

Figure 9.1 Clonal progress in colo-rectal cancer. Predominant (but not exclusive) sequence of evolutionary events in colo-rectal cancer illustrated in terms of changes visualized by conventional histopathology (left) in parallel with identified molecular genetic changes (right). This diagram considerably underplays the complexity of molecular evolution in colo-rectal cancer. For those thirsty for more detail, see the authoritative review by Ilas M, Straub J, Tomlinson IPM and Bodmer WF (1999) *Eur J Cancer*, 35: 335–351.

In some tissue biopsies, it has been possible to 'catch' the dominant invasive subclone emerging from a background of the more benign parental clone. Molecular genetic comparison of the two clones then identifies what mutations are shared (and therefore relatively early acquisitions) and those that are found only in the invasive subclone (and therefore later arrivals). This type of evaluation endorses the credibility of putative evolutionary sequences that are constructed by aligning separate snapshots of the process.

This seems straightforward enough. However detailed molecular profiling of serial samples from individual patients over a period of several years reveals more complex and interesting evolutionary patterns.[10] In unique circumstances, it is possible to study the dynamics of histopathological and molecular evolution of premalignant clones, over time, in individual patients. Superficial bronchial tree lesions can be visualized by a method called fluorescence bronchoscopy and then sampled by biopsy. A small sample of Canadian patients who were heavy smokers and therefore at risk of bronchial carcinoma were investigated. In general, the study confirmed that the more advanced the lesion in terms of histopathological grade, the more genetic lesions were found. More particularly, in six patients who were serially assessed over a two-year period, individual lesions either regressed (in three cases), persisted (four cases) or advanced (one case) with a concordant change or persistence in molecular profile.

In another recent study, it was possible to conduct a detailed molecular scrutiny over time (around six years) of clonal descendants in cancers evolving in the oesophageal epithelium of serially biopsied individual patients. This again confirmed that the overtly cancerous cells usually had higher complements of genetic abnormalities. What it also revealed is the remarkable degree of diversity of subclones within the master or parental clone, each apparently following divergent evolutionary routes in terms of mutational spectrum.

A clear implication of studies such as these is that the evolutionary tree of each patient's cancer clone has a complex branching pattern or clonal population structure which, in detail, is unique to that patient. The evolutionary pathways to success for cancer clones are therefore not fixed or predictable linear progressions, although a time sequence of pathology snapshots or incomplete molecular profiles provide the illusion that they are.[11] Common constellations of mutations and ordered accumulation may indeed occur within dominant cancer clones but the evolutionary route map is not preordained. Neither should we expect it to be. This previously unappreciated layer of molecular complexity has important implications for clinical prognostication and selection of optimum therapy.

Go, stop, go?

The evolutionary patterns of cancer clones that have now been revealed have interesting and provocative implications for our understanding of the natural history of the disease(s). Interrogating normal tissues of adults for histological or molecular signatures of cancerous clones has provided insights that initially are both surprising and alarming but on reflection are neither. Skin on exposed parts of our body in normal adults has around 50 clones with mutant *p53* per square centimetre (each clone being composed of around 60 to 3000 cells). Our faces and hands may have thousands in total. But clearly the odds are very much against any of these clones evolving to cause trouble. As we move into our fifth decade, most of us will have clonal polyps that are signatures of the first steps along the tortuous road to cellular emancipation. Fortunately, at each step of the way, fewer make it. If you ask then, what was different about the patient with colon cancer, then part of the answer appears to be that more aberrant crypts start off the journey – which most likely shifts the odds of one completing the trip.

The same applies to the natural history of prostate and breast cancer. Most ageing men (say, 70 years plus) have a locally invasive carcinoma as revealed by autopsy studies on prostate glands in individuals who died of non-malignant causes. Similarly for breast cancer. The lifetime risk of carcinoma *in situ* (CIS) – a halfway house in cancer development – in the breast may be as high as one in four. In one so far unconfirmed Danish study of biopsies from medico-legal autopsies, one third of women in their 40s had CIS and around half of these were multifocal or bilateral. None were found in a small sample of women in their 20s. Quite possibly, with molecular probes for mutant geno-types, we might well find that the majority of females aged 30 to 50 have these occult clonal incursions or mini-cancers on hold with one or two mutant cards, but falling short, well short perhaps, of the full set required for causing trouble. And clearly the majority of these will never in a lifetime collect a full house of mutations and so graduate to overt and invasive cancers. What then is different about the individuals whose prostates or breasts go on to develop fully fledged cancer? Here, it doesn't look like only a matter of the number of 'starters' but also something that alters the probability of completing the evolutionary trip. Chance? Noxious exposures? Or both? Clearly, the implica-tions of these findings for understanding both the natural history and causality of cancers are considerable. In particular, they reveal that cancer is not the all or nothing phenomenon we might have imagined it to be.

The widespread presence of covert mini- or precancerous lesions in healthy individuals finds a parallel in other chronic diseases that are common in developed societies and that reach their apogee in older age. Post-mortem examination of young adults in their 20s in Europe and the USA has revealed a very high incidence of coronary artery atherosclerotic plaques – between one third and two thirds of all individuals studied. Higher levels during adulthood (25–64 years) have been found in relation to cigarette smoking. We are playing dangerous games and are fortunate that our bodies are so robust.

The evolutionary process of cancer clone development is not only an inefficient and uncertain process but a very protracted one involving a preclinical phase, sometimes referred to as latency, and a progressive history after diagnosis if therapy is unsuccessful. During periods of dormancy, some cancer cells may literally be sleeping, out of the proliferative cycle and in metabolic slumber. But recent insights into the dynamics of cancer clone evolution also indicate that apparent dormancy, in micrometastases for example, persists because of a stand-off between proliferation and cell death. This precarious balance is usually breached when angiogenesis clicks in and growth is facilitated.

A simple, time-ordered sequence can disguise great variability in dynamics. Progression towards a full house is very unlikely to occur at a steady pace. Rather, what happens is more a chaotic, staccato, and unpredictable competitive game with bottlenecks, decimation, long periods of stasis or dormancy, and field days of expansion for individual clones or subclones within the master clone – again very much akin to diversification of species. The consequence of this essential evolutionary feature is that most cancers probably develop with very variable or non-linear dynamics that include irregular steps or jumps (waves of clonal selection and expansion) spread over time periods that can vary from days to decades. The process, once started, is unending in the absence of effective treatment – with a clear evolutionary parallel to both species diversification in general and parasite adaptation.

For most of the common adult cancers, we know that evolution of a benign tumour to its highly metastatic and malignant subclone, or the interval between the initiation of an emergent clone and a diagnosis of cancer, takes many years and usually several decades. For much of this period, the process is covert, clinically silent, and, in a sense, benign. For how long does the clock tick? There are infrequent but instructive situations where cancer follows a point source or acute exposure to a known carcinogen such as the atomic bomb in 1945 in Japan or in patients developing cancer following therapeutic exposure to carcinogenic drugs or irradiation. In these situations, the shortest known interval between exposure and cancer (leukaemia in these cases) is around 18 months but for most leukaemias and especially for the common solid cancers such as breast carcinoma, the interval is 5 to 30 years, depending upon age at exposure and dose.

Since the majority of our cancers do not involve recognized acute initiation but rather chronic, sustained insults, we have less secure insight into the evolutionary time frames involved. Even so, it is clear that it is almost invariably very protracted. Prospective monitoring of patients with benign tumours or growths, for example breast tumours, intestinal polyps, or skin warts, that eventually progressed into florid cancers indicate that intervals of 10–20 years are common. For cancers historically associated with chronic industrial exposures to carcinogenic substances such as coal tars and oils or asbestos, the interval between first exposure and cancer has usually been more than 25 years and often 40 or 50 years. Similarly for cigarette smoking. Of course in these situations, we usually have no way of knowing when the first mutation initiating clonal evolution actually occurred. Epidemiological evidence in melanoma and breast cancer suggests that cancers commonly appearing at around 45–55 years of age can be initiated in the teenage years. Finally, animal experiments have demonstrated that a chemically initiated but stalled cancer clone can hover with malignant intent for most of the life of the animal.

Clonal evolution normally accelerates as the cancer clone successfully metastasizes to many sites, especially if treatment is unsuccessful. But in cases where the disease is effectively controlled, relapses or re-emergence of the same cancer clone (or a mutant subclone thereof) can sometimes occur after 10 to 25 years of silence. This profound dislocation in time and the lack of predictability of the process does much to frustrate both the study of cancer in patients and its effective management. The fact that many cancers silently diversify and disseminate from their site of origin before precipitating diagnostic symptoms is the major reason for treatment failure and mortality. In this respect, some cancers, including those of the ovary, pancreas, and lung, are more stealth-like in their behaviour than others. This fatal time lag must also tangibly influence many people's perception of causation and intuitive weighing of risk. Hazardous sports and lotteries and a host of other activities have primed us to expect risks to be closely coupled in time with rewards or penalties. This, despite us being the only species with the ability to contemplate the future.

Even when apparently well down the evolutionary route to malignancy cancerous cells can occasionally regress or spontaneously vanish. This happens more often with some types of cancer than others, including kidney cancers and melanoma, where credit to our immune defences may be due. In most cases however they are, cruelly, only kidding and cancer returns with a vengeance. But sometimes they really do seem to spontaneously snuff it. This remarkable reprieve has something of a historical precedent. In the thirteenth century, a young priest had cancer in his leg (osteosarcoma?) and was due for an amputation the next day. Miraculously, his fervent prayers the night before the surgeon's knife resulted in a dramatic cure the next morning. Canonized centuries later as St Peregrine, our fortunate patient was content in the knowledge that divine intervention enabled him to live to be 80. The story is no doubt apocryphal but the fact is that a small minority of cancers do regress to the point that we cannot see them. Patients have their own explanations but scientists as yet do not. But it's just a matter of time. Still, if you prefer a more mystical solution then you should know that St Peregrine has become the official patron saint for cancer sufferers. You can find a shrine to him in a grotto at the Old Mission San Juan Capistrano in California. Testimonies to the apparent curative power of prayers are on display.

CHAPTER 10

GREEN-EYED
MUTATIONS?

U p until now, I've talked somewhat glibly about mutant genes in cancer cells as if identifying them and understanding their function in enabling clonal evolution has been a straightforward task. In fact it has taken little less than a technological revolution and intellectual *tour de force* by the biomedical research community to reach this point. Much of this progress has been skilfully chronicled elsewhere by the pilgrims involved. Identifying individual mutant genes has important implications, not only for unravelling the evolutionary process of cancer clone development but for sensitive and differential diagnosis, prognostication, monitoring of residual or cryptic disease, and possibly treatment. You don't need here a catalogue of the hundreds of genes involved but a little insight into the nature of these mutations will help reinforce the evolutionary thread of this story and hopefully convince you that molecules indicted as culprits at one critical level in the causal pathway for cancer have been well and truly fingered.

Until relatively recently, most of the changes to DNA in cancer cells were invisible or submicroscopic. An important exception however are those mutations that involve major or gross changes in chromosome structure or number. Figure 10.1 is one simple and visual example (a leukaemic cell with an additional copy of one of its chromosomes). Altered numbers of chromosomes in cancer cells have been observed for around a hundred years and their causal significance predicted by Boveri, but identifying the particular chromosomes involved and visualizing structural changes has been relatively more recent. Structurally altered chromosomes were first recorded in the early 1960s, in leukaemia, and as the inventory of these increased, it became clear to Janet Rowley in Chicago, and a few other pioneers in the field, that the consistent association of particular structural abnormalities with particular cancers was providing chromosome landmarks for the localization of the pertinent, or impertinent, genes involved. Advances in gene cloning and fine gene mapping on chromosomes have subsequently provided the archaeological tools for uncovering the molecular anatomy of these DNA defects – one of the major discoveries of twentieth-century biomedicine.

At a mechanistic level, mutations in genes leading to cancer can take many structural forms. The most subtle are single-letter changes in the DNA code altering one amino acid unit in the resultant protein which, in turn, is altered in its molecular connectivity to other signals. As a consequence, the protein may, for example, be rendered blind to a restraining signal and hence persistently active. More substantial physical changes include small- or large-scale loss (deletions) of DNA, extra copies (amplifications) of genes, and gains or losses of whole chromosomes.

Loss of genetic information is generally regarded as a mechanically 'simple' way of providing selective advantage to a cell by discarding or dumping genes that encode critical restraining functions, though both parental copies of such a negatively acting gene may have to be lost. Alternatively, and as often happens, one mutated copy may not only lose its normal inhibitory function but interfere with the activity of the remaining normal copy. The end result is the same: loss of some critical restraining function. Extra copies of genes, or whole chromosomes, are somewhat more of a puzzle, but a plausible explanation for their currency in cancer is that the extra copies of one or more proteins that ensue can intercede as decoys in signal relays quenching or diverting incoming messages soliciting compliant responses. Alternatively, the excess protein may acquire intrinsic signalling ability via self-association – interference, one way or another, of signal relays.

Other mutations in DNA involve relatively gross and dramatic chromosomal gymnastics or rearrangements. These derive from chromosome breakage and aberrant restitching, producing fusion and illegitimate partnership of genes that are normally separate entities on different chromosomes – a shuffling of the genetic pack. The molecular consequence of these genetic liaisons is the execution of a *pas de deux* sending altered signals to the cell. Upstream gene A may compel its new downstream partner to be continually expressed or 'on' (a signal to proliferate), when it should be 'off' and 'on' on demand. Alternatively, the two genes may unite to form a single hybrid gene which can then engender a chimaeric protein with altered functions. Many of these latter fused genes encode proteins that interact physically with DNA and play a critical role in regulating the on/off activity of many other genes; they have 'master' regulatory functions in signal relays within the nucleus. It is not surprising therefore that an alteration in their activity can have profound consequences for a cell's pattern of behaviour.

Mutant hybrid genes of this latter kind are particularly prevalent in leukaemias and sarcomas where they appear to provide a potent block to differentiation and hence sustained immaturity. Mutation by aberrant gene joining in single cells parallels the evolutionary advantage of genetic recombination in fertilized eggs that arises via sexual reproduction and shuffling of parental genomes. It's a rapid means of extending genetic diversity and hence potential survival or reproductive fitness. That genetic shuffling should occur at all is perhaps surprising, although we know that it is an ancient game played by some bacteria, viruses, plant species (maize), and *Drosophila* fruit flies that have mobile genetic elements (commonly referred to in the trade as transposons or jumping genes). It is also the basis upon which our immunological repertoires are constructed at the DNA level. Furthermore, it appears that the biochemical mechanisms involved in illegitimate recombination, or 'cut and paste' of genes, require no novel activity by cancer cells but rather represent misdirection of cellular functions that are part of the normal or physiological control of DNA breakage, rejoining, repair, and recombination.

All of these types of alterations in DNA are also not unique to cancer; they occur not only in other genetic, inherited disorders but are, in principle, the driving force for all biological diversity upon which Darwinian selection operates in nature.

Evidence for the prosecution

How do we know that the mutations we can detect in cancer cells are really the driving force for clonal escape? A parallel argument runs throughout evolutionary biology: how do we know that a particular feature or phenotype (with its underlying genotype) constitutes an adaptive feature with selective value for reproductive success? The 'devil's advocate' view championed by Stephen Jay Gould is that the apparently adaptive feature might not have been selected as such but rather it is either a by-product of some other feature or is just the product of an evolutionary accident. Niles Eldredge champions the same so-called 'naturalist' cause which sees evolution as 'just history' and natural selection as no more than a passive filter. Some features of cancer cells and even some of their mutations could fall within this net, but the consistent mutations and their phenotypic consequences do not. The assumption is that we see them distilled out from the thousands of other mutations that must occur because they endow selective advantage to an emergent clone. But what is the evidence for utility in this context? How do we pin the blame on any particular suspect gene, particularly in the light of our knowledge that a gang will have committed the felony?

The consistency with which particular mutations are selectively associated with certain subtypes of cancers is certainly suspicious, particularly when the same mutation is observed both as an acquired or non-inherited genetic abnormality and also as an inherited gene in families predisposed to the same cancers. Being present and behaving suspiciously (as a mutant) when the crime is committed is certainly incriminating. But this is guilt by association, not direct or damning evidence.

When we take a close look at gene mutations – at the sequence of nucleotide bases in the DNA – we find another marker signifying selective value or criminal potential. The mutations are such as to predictably alter the expression or activity of the protein encoded by the gene, as opposed to neutral mutations that have no functional impact. The latter must occur unless our notions of mutation mechanisms are way off beam, but we don't see them in dominant cancer clones, presumably because they confer no selective value.

A further good test of adaptive function in evolution, as Dan Dennett has argued, is to indulge in some 'reverse' engineering: take a close look at the detailed mechanics and see if they provide a functional logic of good design (for a cancerous cell in this case); and then see if manipulation of those features produces the expected changes in behaviour. In this sense, the biochemical functions of mutant genes in cancer cells constitute highly incriminating evidence of guilt. Once genes that are altered in cancer cells are identified and molecularly cloned (that is, multiple copies made), usually in bacteria, it is a relatively straightforward matter to predict and then determine the biochemical function of the normal protein product encoded by the gene and that of its mutant counterpart. Translating the code sequence of the gene often reveals domains that have known functions in other proteins. If the mutation occurs within a region of a domain that is known from X-ray crystallographic studies to be critical for molecular interactions governing some enzymatic function, then the selective logic of the mutation becomes transparent. We can see then how it is that these mutations can endow reproductive advantage (by disrupting a regulatory signal network and, as a downstream consequence, say inhibiting cell death or neutering a negative regulator of cell growth). This evidence endorses the plausibility of guilt on the part of the accused gene but still falls short of sealing the case.

Definitive proof comes from demonstrating that mutant genes can cause or contribute to cancer. Molecular cloning, genetic engineering, and gene transfer techniques have revolutionized our ability to investigate genes for function – good or bad. But the first such 'experiment' with cancer genes happened by accident. The discovery of the first cancer gene was, as often is the case in science, serendipitous. The Rous sarcoma virus causes cancer in chickens and within the viral genome is one vital gene, required for its malignant potential. This was called *v-src* and the Nobel Prize-winning but unanticipated observation was that this gene was a normal cellular gene of chickens that had been 'stolen' by the virus. Subsequently other viruses of laboratory animals have been found to have hijacked normal cellular genes that, like *SRC*, have critical regulatory functions. When these cellular genes become co-opted into the viral

repertoire, a Trojan horse is created. The virus now promotes its own reproductive advantage in cells it infects by compromising the very same cellular
controls that would be corrupted if the same endogenous gene was mutated in
a cancer cell. The fact that these laboratory viruses cause cancer is in a sense an
accident or by-product of the clever ploy they have adopted to facilitate their
own replication in proliferating cells, but it provides compelling evidence for
the pivotal role of particular genes and their mutant forms in cancer.

The first mutated human cancer gene to be discovered (a *RAS* gene, as in
King Ferranti I) was identified via its ability to induce cancer-like behaviour
after transfer into cells in tissue culture. Even so, this same gene turns up as a
pilfered mutant in some leukaemia viruses of laboratory mice. As you might
expect, the gene transfer type of experiment only works well if the recipient
cells have already incurred one or more hits (contributing to a set). More
persuasively perhaps, the transfer of candidate cancer genes into the germ cells
(fertilized eggs) or early embryos and hence into successive generations (of
rodents not humans) or alternatively knocking them out of the germ cell line,
provides dramatic and convincing evidence of guilt. Depending upon the
particular gene that is transferred or knocked out, and whether the offspring
have a single (heterozygous) or double (homozygous) gene dose, a variable but
usually high number of offspring will either succumb to cancer or be much
more vulnerable to the induction of cancer. And then engineering in two
mutant genes with complementary function is more potent. To be frank, the
experiment is a bit of a cheat as every cell in the body now has the mutant
gene(s), though as we shall see, some cancer patients have started life with
essentially the same genetic burden and cancer risk. The ideal experiment –
sequential construction of the mutant genotype in single cells to convert a
socially respectable cell into a metastasizing vagrant – is rather more tricky. But
it was, in 1999, finally achieved, by Bob Weinberg and his colleagues at M.I.T. in
Boston.[12] The virtuoso experiment involved three genetic tricks that together
corrupted four cellular signalling pathways. The cancerous assembly involved:
(1) 'insertion' of an enzyme to protect chromosome ends and to make cells
potentially immortal; (2) provision of a viral oncogene that can block both *p53*
and a critical cell cycle inhibitor gene (called *Rb*); and (3) insertion of a mutant
RAS gene. Normal human epithelial cells so genetically engineered behave as
disseminating cancer cells (in immunodeficient mice). This isn't quite the
genetic route of cancer evolution in patients but it is a dramatic demonstration
of minimal requirements, a potent endorsement of the impact of corrupting
complementary signal networks and a damning indictment of particular genes
in the causal pathway.

Looking at the evidence in its totality, the verdict must, I submit, be guilty as
charged. A handful of biologists do still believe that there is a credible defence

plea but I am afraid, dear jury member, I consider it too incredible to merit reiteration here. Of course there are mitigating circumstances. Mutant genes aren't *the* cause of cancer any more than they are *the* cause of evolution. Gene mutations or losses are accidents aided or abetted in some cases by noxious exposures and the genetic changes only carry selective value in a particular context; this being within the social dialogues that reverberate through the cell, tissues, and body in which they arise. A kind of innocence I suppose.

Picking a winner

The credentials or rules for a dominant cancer clone are, in principle, straightforward: a full house or complementary set of mutant genes for expansion and bottleneck negotiation plus enough time – a lifetime. But what exactly constitutes a winning genotype (gene set) and phenotype (functional attributes)? It is not a fixed or obvious entity (see Fig. 10.2) despite conservation of the underlying principles and generic prescription. It will be very dependent upon context as well as chance and vary in detail according to the cell type involved, the tissues or organ (ecosystem) being colonized, the patient's age, sex, and physiology, and most certainly by the intervention of the physician with a particular cocktail of toxic therapy. You might have imagined for example that getting out in front by proliferating at a fast pace was the ace card for a cancer cell. Not necessarily so, as in Aesop's hare and tortoise fable. The clone that is fast out of the blocks in the evolutionary race to malignancy does not necessarily pass the winning post first. Statistically speaking, it may be the one to bet on, but other clones that are smaller or that start up later could overtake the front runner if they are the beneficiaries of the mutational lottery.

The race may also be handicapped. Cells selected for very rapid reproduction may gain short-term advantage but could be compromised and die if nutrient supplies in their particular tissue environment become limited. For a cancer cell to successfully metastasize to other sites in the body requires attributes that are independent of proliferation rate – ability to degrade physical barriers in tissues and the toughness or resilience to survive the anoxic conditions, turbulence, or stress that changing environments may entail. Finally, working against the hare is therapy itself – equivalent in evolutionary terms to a major or global ecological disaster such as the postulated giant asteroid strike that led to the demise of the dinosaurs 65 million years ago. Who, within the cancer clone, are the survivors? Not the fast runners who will be more vulnerable to cytotoxic radiation and chemotherapy than any sluggish siblings.

What matters in this bottleneck is survival, pure and simple. So those cells that are taking a rest from proliferation or who have placed effective roadblocks on the cell death pathway or who have infiltrated tissues that provide a sanctuary from drug exposure (such as the central nervous system or testis) will be the more likely beneficiaries of any wholesale clearance. That plus lady luck. Overall, it may pay to move at a more leisurely but persistent pace as long as cell production outstrips loss. When it comes to the major evolutionary bottlenecks, it's not the fastest runners or the previously dominant subclones that necessarily get through. It is therefore paradoxical but not surprising that some slow-growing lymphomas and carcinomas (prostate and some breast cancers for example) are amongst the most malignant and clinically intransigent cancers.

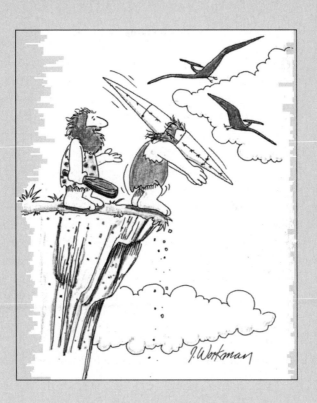

Figure 10.2 'Are you sure about this, Stan? It seems odd that a pointy head and long beak is what makes them fly.'

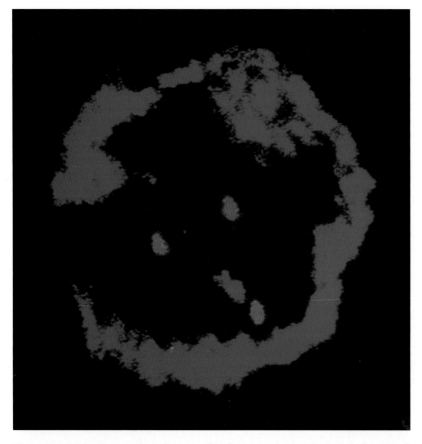

Figure 10.1 Molecular mug shot of cancer cell. A fluorescent image of a single leukaemic cell obtained using a confocal microscope. The three green spots are the result of binding of a DNA probe to chromosome number 8. In a normal cell there would be two copies. In this cancer cell, there are three (as a result of one of the normal copies duplicating). An extra copy of one particular chromosome pair (triploidy) or of several pairs (hyperdiploidy) is one of the more common and simple genetic alterations in cancer, although its functional consequences are not fully understood. The red colour is the result of an antibody binding to the cell cytoplasm. This enables the investigator to know what type of blood cell this leukaemia originates from. The black area inside the red is the cell nucleus.

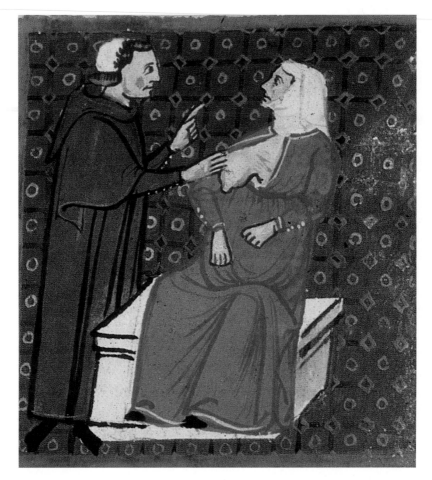

Figure 15.1 Examination of the breast by the surgeon, Teodorico Borgognoni (1275).

CHAPTER 11

OFF TO A SHAKY START

Mutant? Who, me?

Although the majority of mutant genes in cancer arise in single cells in specialized tissues, some cancers involve transmission and inheritance of a mutant gene from parent to offspring. For this to occur requires that at some time in the history of the patient's family one individual predecessor acquired a new mutation in one of his or her germ cells (sperm precursors or ova). Dad's germ cells are more at risk than Mum's because of the greater number of cell divisions that will have occurred prior to conception. We cannot prove how any one such mutation has arisen but most are likely to be accidental consequences of DNA replication, mismanagement, and error-prone repair in germ cells. This seems a thoroughly undesirable and unnatural thing to happen, an appalling lapse of genetic vigilance. But in fact it's part of nature.

The germ line is the sole and critical repository of the genetic information that is relayed between the generations. But its chemically-based code isn't sacrosanct and it cannot be insulated from mutation – not altogether at least. If the spontaneous mutation rate was very high, then for a species such as our own, with modest-sized broods of offspring, we would now be extinct. But a low rate of error or mutation in DNA is both the inevitable consequence of the structure of DNA and its means of replication and a property that holds currency for evolutionary adaptability. The actual rate of error has been engineered by evolutionary forces and is a trade-off between potentially beneficial and harmful effects. We are all mutants. The calculation is that, on average, we inherit around a hundred mutations, newly formed in the sperm and egg from whence we came, in addition to the set of mutations that have been accumulated and passed down the line from grandparents or their ancestors. It's all part of the parental package deal.

Our inherited bank of 30 000 to 40 000 genes is deposited along 23 pairs of chromosomes. So where within this 46-book library are mistakes in copying most likely to occur? It is probably not entirely random. Local topography of DNA may make a difference; big and active genes might be more vulnerable. But most essentially the chance of incurring an unrepaired mutation is entirely unlinked to the biological function encoded in the gene, and hence blind to consequences. Most new mutations will occur in the bulk non-coding or 'junk' DNA that surrounds our genes; others will have neutral effects on genes. But a few will be consequential for our health. And, from time to time, these will include a mutation that can contribute to the emergence of cancerous clones in an offspring. You might suppose that such unwelcome and dangerous genes would be filtered out by natural selection and most probably in the past many have been – if, that is, those with the mutant gene died before they themselves reproduced. The trouble is, however, that such 'bad news' genetics may not always be manifested as disease, say, in the absence of other contributory factors or, if it does produce life-threatening illness, may only do so after reproduction has commenced – after the buck has been passed. Plus, new potentially deleterious mutations will arise anew, at a low rate, in each generation.

Other inherited mutant genes may be recessive in their impact. That's to say that if only one parental copy is mutant or defective, the other non-mutant parental copy may compensate or provide for normal function. In this way, potential harmful genes can travel in the generational train for very many years but only have an impact if an offspring receives a double copy of the mutant (that is, one from each parent). This explains why the most common mutation causing cystic fibrosis has persisted, mostly in silent transit, since it originated in a single individual an estimated 55 000 years ago.

Deleterious gene mutations are therefore historical contingencies and very much part of the natural world – some very ancient, others newly derived. This holds for cancer genes, for unsavoury genes in thalassaemia, cystic fibrosis, and the 5000 or so other inherited genetic disorders that we would rather do without.

One obvious consequence of these historical genetic mishaps is that cancers may be more prevalent in families of related individuals. Familial cancer has been suspected for centuries and clearly recognized and documented for more than a hundred years in the form of pedigrees that defy statistical odds of chance conglomerations. Figure 11.1 illustrates the family tree of a Madame Z in which a large number of descendants had breast or other cancers. This remarkable pedigree covering four generations was the first large cancer family tree to be reported, by surgeon Dr Paul Broca in France in 1852. Most commentators believed that it was his wife's family.

The French have always suspected that the perfidious English killed Napoleon Bonaparte, by poisoning. The Emperor himself lamented that the foul climate on the isolated island of St Helena and the 'English oligarchy and their hired assassins' were responsible for his imminent demise. But Napoleon also knew that cancer could be inherited and in his last months of exacerbating illness, he was convinced that, like his father before him, he too was dying of gastric cancer. He ordered that an autopsy be carried out immediately after his

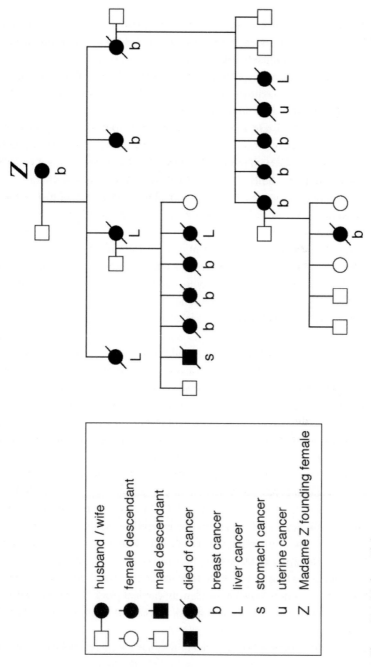

Figure 11.1 Madame Z's legacy.

death in order that this could be confirmed. The report was to be for the benefit of his son, in the hope that it might help him to avoid the disease. In the event the autopsy was performed, on Napoleon's billiard table, by his Corsican doctor, Antommarchi, aided by Scottish naval surgeon, Archibald Arnott. Several other British military surgeons and physicians were in attendance but under instructions from Napoleon that no English hands should touch his body. Their published reports are explicit on the cancerous nature of the lesions found in Napoleon's stomach.

One of Napoleon's sisters, Caroline, also had confirmed gastric cancer and a similar cause of death was suspected for not only his father but also his grand-father, one brother, and two other sisters (see Fig. 11.2)[13] This familial pattern of demise cannot be readily attributed to chance or shared idiosyncrasies in diet. It is very likely therefore that Napoleon, along with several of his siblings, was passed a mutant buck by his father, who in turn acquired his from his father, and so on back.

It is quite likely that in most types of cancer, a minority of cases get kick-started by inheritance of a mutant gene. In some common cancers (including breast, colon, ovary, prostate, melanoma, and thyroid) between 5 and 10 per cent of cases may involve inherited mutations. Family pedigrees with an excess of cancers have provided invaluable material for identification of the genes involved. We will hear more of two of these genes contributing to breast cancer later. But not all cancers that involve an inherited mutant gene are associated with a striking family history. Unless a mutant gene conveys a high risk of cancer of the same cancer type, or is associated with a syndrome of multiple cancer types, it may well not register as genetic predisposition. Also, as new mutations arise all the time (albeit at a low rate) in the germ line, to be inadvertently passed on *de novo* to offspring, some such cancers appear out of the blue, with no prior familial imprint or warning signs.

It is however a relatively straightforward technical matter to test whether a mutant cancer gene has an inherited origin or not. If it has, it will be constitutive (that is, in every cell of the body) rather than being restricted to the cancer clone. For several of such inherited genes investigated, only about half are associated with an unambiguous familial clustering of cases. Around one half of the kick-started cancers may therefore involve new mutations. With molecular identification of the mutant genes involved and armed with some family history, it is now possible to identify carriers prior to onset of illness, raising prospects for genetic screening, risk assessment, monitoring, and early intervention.

Some of the inherited genes involved in familial cancer regulate DNA repair or the detection of DNA damage. A potential consequence of inheriting a mutant variety of one of these genes is global genetic instability in cells and a

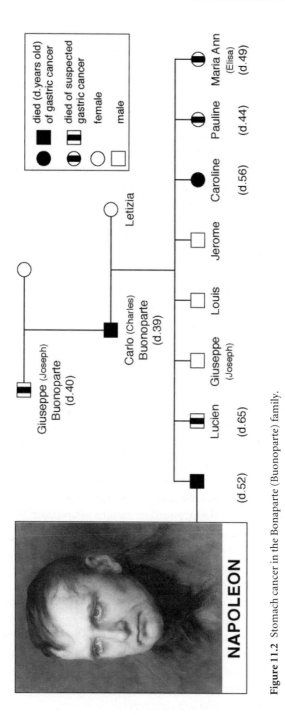

Figure 11.2 Stomach cancer in the Bonaparte (Buonoparte) family.

very high risk of cancer, including a risk of more than one type of cancer or even simultaneous cancers, and at a relatively young age. This is alarming but more or less what you would expect of genes when the evolutionary accelerator function is usurped by mutation. The actual risk will depend also on the functional impact of the individual mutation and whether there is or is not a normal parental copy of the same gene that can compensate for or neutralize the impact of the mutant copy. A mutant *p53* gene in the germ line, for example, is bad news. Individuals with so-called Li-Fraumeni syndrome inherit a single mutant *p53* gene from one or other parent and with it a heightened, though not inevitable, risk of osteosarcomas, breast, and other cancers.

One remarkable insight here and in other cancer syndromes was the realization that the very *same* gene mutation can be involved in cancer either as an inherited or constitutive abnormality present in every cell *or* independently acquired in a single specialized cell type. The difference being that the former is much more likely to lead to cancer.

In a sense, the individual who inherits, via his or her parental lottery, a mutant cancer gene is 'primed' for cancer or strongly predisposed. The evolutionary process of cancer development will involve not one but very many candidate clones. In one form of hereditary colon cancer for example, multiple independent primary tumours or polyps, each a clone, can form in such profusion (many thousands) that critical second or subsequent mutation strikes leading to full-blown cancer are virtually inevitable. In contrast, when the same mutant gene, called *APC*, arrives not via the fertilized egg but in a single colon stem cell, then the chances of progression to cancer are considerably less. But the only invariant rule in cancer biology is that once you establish a firm rule, it's broken. To the chagrin of most sleuths in breast cancer genetics, it came as a surprise that the now famous *BRCA1* and *BRCA2* genes, responsible for (some of) the familial predisposition to breast cancer, were found not to be involved as acquired mutations in 'sporadic' or non-inherited breast cancer.

The inherited mutant cancer genes identified so far convey a high risk to the carrier but in fact account for only a minority of familial cases. It is very likely therefore that other mutant genes, lurking in the germ line, remain to be discovered. Some of these may in themselves carry a lower risk and are referred to by geneticists as being 'less penetrant'. For technical reasons, these genes are more difficult to identify in a family setting and we have no accurate estimation of their number. However, as mutants, such genes, whether highly or poorly penetrant, impact directly on the clonal evolution of cancer cells. The odd but very interesting exception being a mutant that corrupts tissue environment in a way that encourages cancer cell emergence.[14]

There are very many other inherited genes that, though not usually regarded as mutant or abnormal, also impact on cancer, but indirectly. They modify risk and are important because they are widespread in the population. They exist as normal but alternative forms with variable gene sequences and, as a result, variable levels of function. As a consequence of the parental lottery, we all inherit sets of these genes that modify some risks up, and some down.

The genetic package deal

Two of these sets in particular appear to participate in the network of factors that modify the potential impact of cancerous exposures. This they do by modulating the effective dose or level of insult to DNA. These genes have some evolutionary antiquity and the logic of their function and adaptive value is now reasonably transparent. One set are the HLA or histocompatibility genes residing in a cluster on chromosome pair number 6. These are a complex set of multiple genes encoding cell surface proteins identified in the context of tissue or organ transplantation. The genes and the products they encode exist in multiple variations (called polymorphisms or alleles) in all outbred populations. The reason that this extensive natural variation in the gene code sequence and its products exists is that the HLA proteins play a critical role in interaction with alien microbes and, in effect, help 'present' foreign shapes to the immune system. Hypervariability in HLA proteins then contributes to the versatility and specificity of immune recognition and surveillance. We all have a different repertoire in this respect, though identical twins will be the same and siblings have a one in four chance of inheriting the same set of genes. The reason this matters is that as several types of cancer involve persistent infection with viruses, it is very likely that, as with any microbial infection, some of us, by accidental virtue of our particular HLA variants, will be endowed with an immune system that is more or less efficacious at dealing with that particular bug.

Other sets of genes we all inherit in variant forms impact on DNA exposure to chemical carcinogens. We have evolved in a biosphere replete with natural chemical toxins, many of which, in plants for example, exist to warn and ward off potential predators. A very early evolutionary adaptation of animal cells was therefore to develop biochemical mechanisms that could neutralize or detoxify any potentially offensive chemical that arrives via the diet. Some hundreds of genes subserve this protective process in human cells and underscore its importance. It operates via a cascade of enzyme reactions, the most well-known components of which are called cytochrome p450s. These eventually degrade or neuter the offending molecule though paradoxically, at the beginning of the chain reaction, some molecules are transiently activated to become more carcinogenic. These enzymes and the genes that encode them also exist in variant forms. As a consequence and depending upon our inherited maternal and paternal gene sets, we may be better or worse off than the average for handling any assault by a chemical that has DNA-damaging potential. And this may or may not have an impact on health and cancer. It does explain why individuals whose cells are, from the perspective of chemical machinery, 'slow acetylators', may be more at risk of bladder cancers if exposed to certain carcinogenic chemicals. And similarly, why individuals less able to detoxify fungal aflatoxins are more at risk of liver cancer if their liver has also been exposed to and damaged by hepatitis B virus. This pattern of genetics, in other words, combines with other factors in determining the risk of cancer.

Variation in other normal genes probably modifies cancer risk indirectly, for example, genes whose products control repair of DNA damage or participate in hormone signal relays influencing cell proliferation and survival. We are therefore all subject to a double genetic lottery at conception with respect to cancer risk: the presence or absence of mutant cancer genes and the presence of normal gene sets whose intrinsic variation indirectly modifies risk. How much weight should we give to this genetic burden? Does it mean that from birth we are predestined to have, or not have, particular cancers? Certainly the genetically prescribed odds are not equal in all of us, as indeed they probably are not for any ailment that can afflict our species. Some geneticists create the impression, deliberately or not, that the gene is omnipotent and that if we had complete DNA profiles, we could predict who would get what cancer. This is genetic determinism and, as such, cancer is invited to join infidelity, obesity, and ability to do crosswords in a facile portrayal of what we are. I don't know if anyone who understands genetics and biology really believes this. Inherited mutant genes do carry some predictive value, albeit not accurately quantifiable, and it would be interesting and potentially of benefit to have a full catalogue of these. Cancer certainly does evolve in the context of our individual genetic backgrounds and this does matter. But the underlying genetics is complex, multifactorial, and it certainly isn't all.

The risk of getting cancer is a composite or mosaic of inherited genetics, exposure patterns, other modifying activities (diet, for example), and, inevitably, chance. And for this cocktail, we are not yet smart enough to produce a reliable algorithm that allows us to accurately compute actual risk. We will not understand the causation of cancer without taking this complexity on board and without taking the trouble to construct the networks that collectively call the tune. At the end of the day, however, what will matter most is identifying which component in the pathway offers the most practical and effective route for control. And, following this diatribe on molecular mayhem in cancer cells, you may, or may not concur if I venture the opinion that practical control in the future is very unlikely to involve the manipulation of genes.

CHAPTER 12

BLIND CHANCE – AND ULTIMATE EXTINCTION?

Like all evolutionary changes with the appearance of prudent planning or a smart, selfish manoeuvre, cancer cells and their mutations are not strategic by design or intent. They operate by a throwing of the genetic dice at random or by blind chance, coupled with selection for what might be relatively short-term advantage. The process may have all the attributes of a covert collaboration of mutant genes, but in reality it's cock-up and chaos that apply, not conspiracy.

The vast majority of mutations in precancer or cancer cells never see the light of day: nearly all cancer cells die. However, given sufficient numbers of cells and aided, in some cases, by instability in DNA, they can adapt rapidly to a sustained environmental challenge provided by the body's physiological constraints or by cancer therapy. Ultimately, if they succeed in dissemination and resist all therapy, they destroy their only environment – the patient. Dumb parasites? You may be surprised. Given the chance, cancer cells behave as smart parasites revealing both their immortality as a replicating clone and their ability to colonize new hosts. In so doing, cancer cells exploit some ancient evolutionary adaptations.

Going for ever

A cell culture called the HeLa cell line is ubiquitous in cancer research laboratories. It originated from a patient, Henrietta Lacks, who died of cervical cancer more than 40 years ago and, through the efforts of her family, has recently become something of a *cause célèbre* in black America. Her cells are still going strong – too strong. These cells have been not only an important research resource but a nuisance, since they seem to be adept at getting into and taking over other cell cultures kept in the same laboratory. Vigorous growth and sloppy technique rather than wings are however to blame.

The HeLa cell line is not however an exception. Cancer cells taken from patients with relapsed or metastatic disease can now be maintained with sustained proliferation, in test tubes, in perpetuity. Cancer cell lines derived from rodents have been maintained in culture over periods equivalent to ten or more normal life spans. So it is likely that most cancer cell clones are indeed potentially immortal. This isn't just evasion of imposed or suicidal cell death on command (a regular mutant card for cancer cells) but a more subtle and critical ploy. There is a very interesting current debate on how clonal immortality arises in the context of cancer development. Unicellular organisms and parasites can divide indefinitely; they are effectively immortal as a clonal lineage. But they require a trick to achieve this. It turns out that for mechanical reasons it is very difficult to replicate the ends of chromosomal DNA and, as a consequence, each time a cell divides and copies its DNA, it loses a bit of the end of each chromosome (called a telomere). This progressive 'eating away' serves as a cell division clock, marking the run-down of lifetime such that eventually, the erosion of ends reaches a critical point and the cell dies. This is obviously a serious and ancient fault in the design of linear DNA packaged into chromosomes. It wasn't a problem earlier on with antecedent bacteria that have circular DNA.

This problem was solved very early on in the evolution of unicellular organisms by a gene encoding an enzyme called telomerase, that could replace the missing ends with each round of DNA copying. This enzyme is then ubiquitous in the unicellular world of unlimited potential for replication. Upstairs with worms and men, the same enzyme is found principally in two places – germ cells and cancer cells. The conventional wisdom is that it makes sense for our normal body cells to be subject to a proliferative death clock: fifty rounds then your time is up! This might then be an integral component of both clonal restraint and the natural ageing process. But with the progressive evolution of cancer, there is, as I mentioned earlier, bound to be strong selective advantage for any mutant that succeeds in activating the telomerase gene that every cell has, but which is normally silenced. So it would seem. This may well be correct but I have a problem with it. Why have we retained such an ancient gene for cellular immortality? The standard response to this query is that we need it for our germ cells (the stem cells that generate sperms and eggs in testis and ovary). Our germ cell supply at birth must last a lifetime, or rather a normal reproductive lifetime, and with its chromosomes in pristine condition. All well and good. But if this is correct, then the same might be expected to apply to tissue stem cells, our small stock of which is complete at birth but must also last a lifetime. Blood stem cells in mice can be transferred over more than five generations, indicating that they are extremely long-lived, if not immortal. This suggests the possibility that the prime cellular targets for cancer – our stem cells – may already be equipped for immortality which can be exploited when they convert to cancer. Either way, it may not matter; operationally speaking cancer cells adopt yet one other essential trick – they become immortal with the assistance of telomerase and perhaps with other mutations that overcome inbuilt senescence. They could go on forever, if they had the chance.

Crossing the rubicon

But can cancer cells express that other essential characteristic of unicellular parasites – the ability to colonize new hosts? Surely it's crazy to consider that cancer might be contagious even if the idea has a long historical pedigree and a recent survey found that more than 20 per cent of adult Americans believed that you can catch cancer by contact with patients.

Viruses that contribute to the causal mechanism of some cancers are of course infectious, but this is quite different from the issue of whether cancer cells can, parasite-like, transit from one individual to another, survive, and colonize. Anecdotal evidence has in the past encouraged the view that cancer might be contagious. The seventeenth-century Dutch physician, Nicolaes Tulp, immortalized in Rembrandt's painting 'The Anatomy Lesson', referred to a case of ulcerating breast cancer that was believed to have been transmitted from the patient to her housemaid. The French coined an appropriate phrase ('cancer-à-deux') for the simultaneous presence of penis and cervical cancer in a cohabiting couple and which for a time was thought to reflect a contagious cancer. These coincident cancers were almost certainly due to sexual trans-mission and sharing of a species of papilloma virus, the critical agent for these types of cancer, rather than exchange of cancer cells (see Chapter 17).

There would seem to be two rather obvious and powerful restrictions on the transfer of cancer from one individual to another. The first is the efficacy of the immune system in surveillance against anything foreign, and the second is the lack of any safe passage route that cancer cells could exploit to navigate be-tween individuals. The exceptions that break these anticipated barriers are illuminating and extraordinary.

In 1773, the French scientist, Bernard Peyrilhe, in what is the first recorded attempt to transplant cancer, extracted fluids and cells from a breast cancer and injected them into a dog. Hearing the howls of the dog the housekeeper is said to have taken pity on it and drowned it. Peyrilhe's experiment would have failed anyway as cancer cells cannot be transplanted between different species – they are recognized as foreign invaders and rejected, as would be normal cells or tissues. Almost a century ago, it was accepted that cancer cells could be reproducibly transplanted within a species providing the donor and recipient were inbred. Rodent cancer cells can be easily transplanted indefinitely within an inbred strain and human cancer cells will colonize, long-term, mice that have profound immune deficiency.

Human cancer clones would almost certainly develop a parasitic propensity to spread to other individuals if we were not genetically outbred with a versatile and efficacious immune system. The immune system was probably not 'designed' to kill off cancer cells, although this view has been favoured in the past by some very eminent biologists. More probably, it evolved and was credited with selective currency as a mechanism to combat foreign invasion in the form of infection. Any cancer cell coming from you to me, I will immunologically register as alien, foreign, or 'non-me'; potentially offensive and therefore undesirable. If a few cancer cells did pass between individuals, say in body fluids, we would expect them to be immunologically rejected as foreign. If it were not so, history would certainly have recorded otherwise.

In the early part of the nineteenth century, doctors and students at the Hôpital St Louis in Paris inoculated themselves with the discharges of ulcerating cancers without any dramatic consequences. In experiments that would today be regarded as unethical, USA researcher, Chester Southam, showed in the 1960s that cancer cells are indeed rejected or rendered innocuous when deliberately injected into healthy volunteers. To quote:

> ... for this knowledge we are greatly indebted to the prisoners of Ohio State Penitentiary who freely volunteered, without payment or special consideration of any kind, to serve as healthy recipients in this research.

Southam also showed however that transplanted cancer cells would grow, at least as nodules, if the recipient was a cancer patient himself and in an advanced state of illness (and presumably immunosuppressed).

A similar cavalier experiment in the early 1960s did result in the propagation of cancer cells from one individual to another. A melanoma sample from a terminally ill 50-year-old woman was transplanted into the buttock or rectus muscle of her 80-year-old mother in, so it is stated, an attempt to understand cancer immunity. The mother was informed that the tumour from her daughter might grow and metastasize in her own body but the investigators considered the risk of this occurrence very remote. We can only guess at this old lady's judgement at the time. The implanted melanoma biopsy was surgically removed after 24 days but too late to stop its spread. Fifteen months later, the mother died of disseminated melanoma. Melanoma cells are notoriously adept at metastasizing, but the authors of this extraordinary case report offered no insight or thought on why, contrary to their prior firm conviction, dissemination occurred in this case. Mother and daughter did have very similar blood groups so a minimal genetic mismatch might have existed. Additionally, the immune system of an 80-year-old woman might well be less proficient at rejecting alien cells. Either way, this tragic case of a mother dying from her daughter's cancer illustrates that cancer cells can express a remarkable ability to colonize a second individual, when provided with an artificial access route.

Along similar but rather more innocent lines, some immunosuppressed transplant recipients have in the past developed cancer originating from donor cells in the transplanted organ itself. The Cincinnati Transplant Tumor Registry, as of 1991, recorded some 72 patients, mostly kidney recipients, who developed either localized or metastatic cancer soon after transplantation or within three years of a transplant. A variety of cancer types were inadvertently transferred from donors to recipients in this way including lung, kidney, melanoma, and breast cancers. In all these cases, the cancer cells were passively transferred along with the organ and its blood supply to a new host environment where the enforced absence of an active immune system permitted their alien origin, along with that of the beneficial organ graft itself, to go unchecked. These cases represent a tiny fraction of the hundred thousand or more organ transplants performed and almost all occurred at a time more than 30 years ago when the risk of using recently deceased donors who had cancer as providers of organs to immunosuppressed recipients was not appreciated or where the cause of death in the donor was misdiagnosed.

These examples illustrate that although the immune system provides a formidable barrier to cancer cells, it can, albeit under special or facilitated circumstances, be breached. One might even expect it to happen more often. Why, for example, if cancer clones are subject to genetic diversification and intense selective pressure, don't we see emergence of cancer cells that have adopted the trick employed by many parasites? This is the well-worked routine of cloaking the cell in anonymity and is achieved by turning off or covering up molecules that can be recognized as alien. Well, this does in fact happen in cancer. Paradoxically, the first cancer to be successfully transplanted in the 1880s also transplants itself via sexual contact. Venereal sarcoma affects the external genitalia of dogs and has been recognized for over a hundred years as a contagious cancer. Exactly how transmission succeeds isn't entirely clear since the transfer can occur not only between different strains of dogs but, experimentally, from dogs to foxes. What appears to be crucial however is that the sarcoma cells have lost most of the cell surface molecules that identify them as part of an individual dog. In this case at least, intrinsic or genetic foreignness is effectively disguised, an ancient parasite trick effectively adopted.

In the case of human cancer cells, an equivalent scenario would have to involve the so-called histocompatibility or HLA proteins which provide the major molecular discrimination between each of us. Interestingly, cancer cells do in some circumstances downregulate their expression of these cellular flags of identity. This outcome probably derives from situations where the patient's own immune system is activated and selective pressure then facilitates the outgrowth of HLA-negative variants or mutants. But there is no evidence that such cryptic cancer clones can be contagious.

Perhaps the real barrier to contagious cancer cells is the lack of any natural transit route that at least a few cancer cells might navigate. Parasites have evolved to accomplish this feat by exploiting blood-sucking insect vectors or by adopting life cycles that include a very robust extracorporeal stage (muddy waters and the like). This, we presume, took a few million years of trial-and-error evolution. It is asking a lot for cancer cells to achieve this much – even with the mutation accelerator at full throttle.

Despite this apparently insurmountable barrier, there are several remarkable examples of natural cancer cell transfer in humans. These all exploit a unique feature of mammalian evolution – the placenta. The first is a relatively rare form of cancer in women called choriocarcinoma. This cancer is, in effect, a pregnancy gone wrong. The cancer cells derive from a fertilized egg and would normally form the foetal trophoblast tissue which provides the intimate contact zone in the placenta between the developing embryo and its mother's uterus. Abnormal development can take the form of a mole (hydatiform mole) or a frank cancer (choriocarcinoma) that may spread, usually to the lung. Genetically, the cancer cells are foreign in the same sense that a foetus or baby is itself foreign in the womb, although curiously many hydatiform moles and choriocarcinoma have only paternal or father's chromosomes. How then can they invade and metastasize in an alien environment, parasiting the host mother? There are two reasons for this and both reflect sound evolutionary adaptive principles, in this case exclusive to mammalian development. Firstly, normal embryonic trophoblast cells must have invasive capability to carry out their prescribed function in pregnancy (implantation of the embryo in the wall of the uterus). There is biochemical evidence that they use the same or similar mechanisms to invade as, say, breast cancer cells. Indeed some normal embryo trophoblast cells do migrate into the blood circulation of healthy mothers but this process is largely constrained within the placenta. Secondly, the trophoblast cells, though genetically foreign, represent a crucial immunological filter or barrier between the mother and her unborn baby. Without this barrier, the developing foetus would itself be rejected, perceived immunologically as a foreign body or pseudo-infection. In order to exercise this critical function in mammals, trophoblast cells express unique cell-surface properties that render them invisible to the immune system. In addition, recent research suggests that they may secrete an enzyme that comprises the immunological competence of maternal immune cells or lymphocytes. The adaptive logic here is clear but this invisibility has unfortunate consequences if these cells migrate into mother's blood *and* if a clone of them has acquired genetic changes that enable it to colonize and grow in a distant site such as the lung. Fortunately, this is rare (around 1 in 30 000 pregnancies), although for unknown reasons more common in less developed countries.

Choriocarcinoma also provides what is probably the most startling example of parasite-like dissemination between individuals. A few years ago, a 27-year-old woman in Belgium died of a brain haemorrhage and her heart, plus lung, liver, and right kidney were transplanted into three recipients. All three then developed metastatic choriocarcinoma. Two of the recipients were male and there can be little doubt that the cancer came via the female donor organs. The donor herself was thought to have died as a consequence of a rupture in a malformed cerebral blood vessel but, in retrospect, the haemorrhage was probably caused by infiltrating cancer cells. This grim story is paralleled by other similar cases of choriocarcinoma transfer recorded in the Cincinnati Transplant Tumor Registry. It reveals then the most bizarre, improbable, and unfortunate of cancer cell journeys: from foetal tissue to mother and then to other unrelated individuals. On the good news side, choriocarcinoma is remarkably sensitive to chemotherapy and curable in most cases. It was in fact the first metastatic or disseminated cancer to be curable and the reason for this has much to do with its unusual biology, as I shall discuss later.

The second example of parasitization by cancer cells is equally remarkable, doubly tragic, and again involves mishaps during pregnancy. This is when both twins in an identical pair of children suffer from leukaemia. Francis Galton, founder of eugenics and cousin to Charles Darwin, was the first to propose, in 1876, that the comparison of identical and non-identical twin siblings would help distinguish the impact of nature and nurture on an individual's characteristics. It is now well recognized that identical twins are more likely than fraternal or non-identical twins to share the same features, including not only normal physical appearance but numerous psychological traits, cognitive ability, obesity, and diseases such as insulin-dependent diabetes and multiple sclerosis. Similarly, your risk of cancer of the prostate, breast, colon, or cervix is greater if you already have an identical twin (rather than a non-identical twin) with that cancer. Such is the pervasive influence of genes, though sharing of the same inherited gene set in identical twins by no means guarantees sharing or concordance of illnesses or causes of death. Still, you might now guess that leukaemia in identical twins must arise as a consequence of both twins inheriting the same abnormal cancer-predisposing gene. Not so. It turns out that what actually happens is rather more extraordinary: one twin, in effect, catches leukaemia from the other. In my own laboratory, we used molecular methods to show that in several sets of identical twins, the same single mutant clone of leukaemic cells existed in both individuals of each twin pair. The mutation that marked the clone was unique to the pair of twins but at the same time was clearly not inherited. The only plausible explanation for this is that the leukaemic clone originates during pregnancy in one cell in one foetus. Clonal progeny then spread from one to the other twin whilst they are still both in the womb. This is possible because most identical twins share a single placenta with interconnecting blood vessels permitting passage of blood cells. There is no vascular barrier between them as there is between foetus and mother or between non-identical twins with two placentas. But the survival of the parasitic clone must also be dependent upon the fact that it cannot be seen as foreign – coming as it does from an identical twin. Both of the natural barriers to preventing contagious spread are therefore breached in twin leukaemia as in choriocarcinoma. Fortunately again, this type of double cancer is extremely rare.

These cases associated with pregnancy also beg another question. How come the placental barrier isn't breached more often? For example, if a woman with cancer becomes pregnant, why isn't the developing baby vulnerable? Leukaemia might be the obvious example but only two cases have ever been recorded in the newborn offspring of mothers with leukaemia. It is unlikely that the immune system is the saviour in this situation. The foetus has a very immature immune system that should have difficulty in rejecting a maternal cell invasion. The answer is likely to be the evolutionary necessity of a cell-impermeable placental barrier that prohibits transit of maternal immune cells that can reject the foetus as foreign. Prohibition of maternal cancer cell transit is then a fortuitous side-benefit of this early mammalian evolutionary adaptation. Still, some foetal losses or spontaneous abortions have been attributed to immunological rejection and one would expect, very occasionally, cancer cells to smuggle through the placental no man's land and colonize the unborn child. And it does happen, albeit very rarely, with the most imperialistic of cancers – melanoma. At least four cases of cancer spread from pregnant mother to child have been documented. The essential details of one of these cases published more than 60 years ago are as follows: whilst pregnant, the mother had widespread malignant melanoma and had died a few months after the birth of her son. The child was born by Caesarian section and the obstetrician noted that the placenta was huge and black and infiltrated with melanoma. Ten months after birth, the infant boy himself died of melanoma which resided predominantly in the liver but also in other sites. Melanoma in infants is exceedingly rare and in these few unique cases, transfer from mother to her offspring seems very likely to have occurred.

Cancer cells are therefore immortal and parasitic and, under special circumstances, they can be contagious. But don't be alarmed. No cancer scientist has been diagnosed with HeLa cancer and no cancer has been found to transit between conjugal partners or between patient and nurse. Cancer clones evolve fast – but not that fast.

Back to the future

The evolution of cancer clones parallels a marathon obstacle race with many hopeful starters and usually only one winner – if there's a winner at all. Each obstacle is a bottleneck that preferentially lets through the cells with appropriate mutant credentials. Most will trip up or hit the buffers. Winners will have tickets for negotiating or negating hurdles but can be aided and abetted by the normally benevolent processes of tissue repair and re-juvenation. But, as in other evolutionary journeys, the clone that does progress does so without prescience and, symbolically in this case, with no malice aforethought. In effect, the outcome of the cancer cells' travels is a product of its antecedent history and the selective landscapes in which they find themselves. A local landscape or ecosystem that may itself be altered by the presence of a cancer clone, and to the benefit of the instigator.

And at each step of the way, adaptive success is achieved by the fortuitous possession of mutations that can, collectively, deconstruct the interactive networks of signals within and between cells that normally impose com-pliant behaviour. The reproductive imperative becomes progressively un-coupled and insulated from rules for restraint or from penalty clauses. At the point of no return (invasive cancer), a dominant clone emerges with a mutinous character – stone deaf to social dialogue, divorced from its func-tional context, and with its genetic contract eroded. It is immortal and itinerant; free to do nothing but make more of itself. But this character is strangely *déjà vu*. It's back where it started. The obstacle race has been running backwards all along; a resurrection of the long-buried memory of unicellular selfishness. Doing what came naturally, long ago.

NOTES TO PART TWO

1 For example, protozoan unicellular parasites responsible for major illnesses in developing countries, including leishmania, amoebic dysentery, sleeping sickness, and Chagas disease.

2 The idea that cancer cells might be evolutionary revertents is not new. Both Morley Roberts in 1926 and Sir Herbert Snow in 1893 suggested that cancers were derived from cells that retain a memory for amoeba-like selfish behaviour and that can still escape by losing allegiance to the community of cells within which they reside. Roberts' views are scarcely quoted but were remarkably prescient. He saw cancer as a natural evolutionary process and a problem in developmental biology. He recognized that the abilities of some tissues to regenerate under stress and for other cells to migrate and invade provided some of the inherent talent required for cancer cell behaviour. More recently, Lucien Israel has argued that cancer cell emergence might reflect the expression of a cell survival programme originating in our unicellular ancestors and normally put to good use, albeit transiently, in the developing embryo during growth and in wound healing. Israel also contends, however, that the persistent expression of such a programme by cancer cells might not depend upon random mutation and natural selection. See Roberts M (1926) *Malignancy and evolution*, Grayson and Grayson Publishers, London; Snow H (1893) *Cancers and the cancer process*, J and A Churchill Publishers, London; Israel L (1996) Tumour progression: random mutations or an integrated survival response to cellular stress conferred from unicellular organisms, *J Theoret Biol*, **178**:375–80.

3 For a light-hearted but informative romp through the cultural history of skin moles, see Ariel AM (1981) Is the beauty mark a mark of beauty or a potentially dangerous cancer? In: *Malignant melanoma* (chapter one), Appleton-Century-Crofts Publishers, New York.

4 There may be some correlation between the size of polyps and the likelihood of undergoing further evolution towards malignancy. There is no universal rule here however. Benign tumours or polyps can occasionally grow to quite a size without being life-threatening. Bland-Sutton in his book *Tumours: innocent and malignant*, first published in 1893 (Cassells, London), quoted the case of an 'old Welsh woman' with a horn-shaped papillomatous wart some 21cm long.

5 Sometimes referred to as oncogenes and tumour suppresser genes respectively.

6 A much beloved literary quote, already embedded in the lexicon of evolutionary biology. Leigh Van Valen used this as a potent and visual metaphor for evolutionary 'progress': how organisms must be continuously on the move (genetically speaking) and inventive (with sex for example) just to keep pace with parasitic and other competitors who threaten their livelihood. See Matt Ridley's *The Red Queen*, Penguin Group, 1993.

7 The Nobel Prize-winning biochemist, Manfred Eigen, has proposed a similar explanation of the molecular evolution of highly efficient enzymes via serial mutations that are essentially random. In essence, mutants with some superiority over their precursor 'wild type' provide the expanded and exposed venue for further selective forces to operate. Eigen M (1992) *Steps towards life. A perspective on evolution*, Oxford University Press, Oxford.

8 Tomlinson I and Bodmer W (1999) Selection, the mutation rate and cancer: ensuring that the tail does not wag the dog. *Nature Med*, 5:11–12. For a somewhat opposing view on this issue, see Loeb LA (1991) Mutator phenotype may be required for multi-stage carcinogenesis. *Cancer Res*, 51:3075–9.

9 These signalling pathways can be considered as examples of complex adaptive systems incorporating multiple or combinatorial interactions, non-linear dynamics, and novel or emergent properties (behaviour of the stock market is another). Modelling and understanding of such systems is inherently a difficult and complex task, but has been aided by mathematics, chaos theory, and computer simulation. For erudite and lucid exploration of these ideas in the context of cell signalling and cancer, see Schwab ED and Pienta (1997) Explaining aberrations of cell structure and cell signalling in cancer using complex adaptive systems, *Adv Mol Cell Biol*, 24: 207–47; Weng G, Bhalla US, Iyengar R (1999) Complexity in biological signalling systems, *Science*, 284:92–5.

10 See for details: Thiberville L, Payne P, Vielkinds J, LeRiche J, Horsman D, Nouvet G, *et al.* (1995) Evidence of cumulative gene losses with progression of premalignant epithelial lesions to carcinoma of the bronchus. *Cancer Res*, 55:5133–9; and Barrett MT, Sanchez CA, Prevo LJ, Wong DJ, Galipeau PC, Paulson TG, *et al.* (1999) Evolution of neoplastic cell lineages in Barrett oesophagus. *Nature Genet*, 22:106–9.

11 A few astute pathologists recognized this many years ago: Foulds L (1969) *Neoplastic development*, Academic Press, New York.

12 See Hahn WC, Counter CM, Lundberg AS, Beijersbergen RL, Brooks MW,

Weinberg RA (1999) Creation of human tumour cells with defined genetic elements. *Nature*, **400**:464–8.

13 Sources of information: Andrews E (1895) The diseases, death and autopsy of Napoleon I, *J Am Med Assoc*, 1081–5; Sokoloff B (1938) Predisposition to cancer in the Bonaparte family, *Am J Surgery*, **40**:673-8; and Cronig V (1994) *Napoleon*, Harper Collins, London.

14 In these examples of cancerous predisposition, the inherited gene contributes to the aberrant genotype of the cancerous clone, either indirectly by endowing genetic instability and hence risk of further mutation or by directly subverting some intracellular signalling pathway. But other genetic routes to high cancer probability are possible, albeit less frequently observed. For example, in so-called juvenile polyposis syndrome which couples ulcerative colitis with a 10 to 20 per cent likelihood of colonic cancer, the inherited 'defective' gene has its major impact on the cellular environment surrounding the epithelial cells that are at risk of malignant transformation. This has been aptly referred to as a 'landscape' genetic effect. See Kinzler KW and Vogelstein B (1998) *Science*, **280**:1036–7.

FURTHER READING

Historical

Boveri T (1929) *The origin of malignant tumors*. Baillière Tindall & Cox, London – the original, in translation. For a critique see Wolf U (1974) Theodor Boveri and his book 'On the problem of the origin of malignant tumors'. In: German J, ed. *Chromosomes and cancer*. J Wiley, New York.

Lawley PD (1994) Historical origins of current concepts of carcinogenesis. *Adv Cancer Res*, **65**:17–111.

Long ER (1965) *A history of pathology*. Dover Publishers Inc, New York.

Raven RW (1990) *The theory and practice of oncology. Historical evolution and present principles*. The Parthenon Publishing Group, New Jersey.

Clonality in nature

Benditt EP and Benditt JM (1973) Evidence for a monoclonal origin of human atherosclerotic plaques. *Proc Natl Acad Sci USA*, **70**:1753–6.

Cleary PP, Kaplan EL, Handley JP, Wlazlo A, Kim MH, Hauser AR, *et al.* (1992) Clonal basis for resurgency of serious *Streptococcus pyogenes* disease in the 1980s. *Lancet*, **339**:518–21.

da Silva W (1997) On the trail of the lonesome pine. *New Scientist*, **2111**:36–9.

Edelman G (1994) *Bright air, brilliant fire*. Penguin Books, London.

Evolution and development of the body plan

Buss LW (1987) *The evolution of individuality.* Princetown University Press, New Jersey.

Coffey DS (1998) Self-organization, complexity and chaos: the new biology for medicine. *Nature Med*, 4:882–5.

Gerhart J and Kirschner M (1997) *Cells, embryos and evolution.* Blackwell Science, Malden, Massachusetts.

Kauffman SA (1993) *The origin of order. Self-organization and selection in evolution.* Oxford University Press, New York.

Evolutionary biology

Dawkins R (1995) *River out of Eden.* Harper Collins, New York.

Dennett DC (1995) *Darwin's dangerous idea. Evolution and the meanings of life.* Allen Lane, Penguin Press.

Maynard Smith J (1988) *Did Darwin get it right? Essays on games, sex and evolution.* Penguin Books, London.

Williams G (1966) *Adaptation and natural selection. A critique of some current evolutionary thoughts.* Princetown University Press, New Jersey.

Williams G (1996) *Plan and purpose in nature.* Harper Collins, New York.

Cell death

Evan G and Littlewood T (1998) A matter of life and cell death. *Science,* **281**:1317–22 (and other reviews in the same issue of *Science*).

Vaux DL, Haecker G, Strasser A (1994) An evolutionary perspective on apoptosis. *Cell,* **76**: 777–9.

Mutations in nature and as the driving force in cancer

Cairns J (1975) Mutation selection and the natural history of cancer. *Nature,* **255**:197–200.

Eigen M (1992) *Steps towards life. A perspective on evolution.* Oxford University Press.

Jonason AS, Kunala S, Price GJ, Restifo RJ, Spinelli HM, Persing JA, *et al.* (1996) Frequent clones of *p53*-mutated keratinocytes in normal human skin. *Proc Natl Acad Sci USA,* **93**:14025–9.

Sniegowski P (1997) Evolution: setting the mutation rate. *Curr Biol,* 7:487–8.

Vogelstein B and Kinzler KW (1998) *The genetic basis of human cancer.* McGraw-Hill, New York.

Stem cells and developmental origins of cancer

Knudson AG (1992) Stem cell regulation, tissue ontogeny, and oncogenic events. *Sem Cancer Biol*, **3**:99–106.

Pierce GB, Shikes R, Fink LM (1978) *Cancer. A problem of developmental biology*. Prentice-Hall, New Jersey.

Stem cells and regeneration: series of five scholarly reviews. *Science* (1997) pp 60–87.

Clonal evolution of cancer cells

Bodmer WF (1996) The somatic evolution of cancer. The Harveian Oration of 1996. *J Royal College Phys London*, **31**: 82–9.

Burnett M (1974) The biology of cancer. In: German J, ed. *Chromosomes and cancer*. J Wiley, New York, pp 21–38.

Farber E (1973) Carcinogenesis – cellular evolution as a unifying thread: presidential address. *Cancer Res*, **33**:2537–50.

Hopkin K (1996) Tumor evolution: survival of the fittest cells. *J NIH Res*, **8**:37–41.

Nowell PC (1976) The clonal evolution of tumor cell populations. *Science*, **194**:23–8.

Woodruff M, ed. (1990) *Cellular variation and adaptation in cancer*. Oxford University Press, Oxford.

Chromosomal and molecular genetics of cancer cells

Bishop JM (1991) Molecular themes in oncogenesis. *Cell*, **64**:235–48.

Breivik J (2001) Don't stop for repairs in a war zone: Darwinian evolution unites genes and environment in cancer development. *Proc Natl Acad Sci USA*, **98**:5379–81.

Cavenee WK and White RL (1995) The genetic basis of cancer. *Scientific American*, **March**: 50–7.

Hanahan D and Weinberg RA (2000) The hallmarks of cancer. *Cell*, **100**:57–70.

Nowell PC (1993) Chromosomes and cancer: the evolution of an idea. *Adv Cancer Res*, **62**: 1–17.

Sidransky D (1997) Nucleic acid-based methods for the detection of cancer. *Science*, **278**: 1054–8.

Varmus H and Weinberg RA (1993) *Genes and the biology of cancer*. Scientific American Library.

Angiogenesis and metastasis

Kerbel RS (1990) Growth dominance of the metastatic cancer cell: cellular and molecular aspects. *Adv Cancer Res*, **55**:87–132.

Hanahan D and Folkman J (1996) Patterns and emerging mechanisms of the angiogenic switch during tumorigenesis. *Cell*, **86**:353–64.

Liotta LA, Steeg PS, Stetler-Stephenson WG (1991) Cancer metastasis and angiogenesis: an imbalance of positive and negative regulation. *Cell*, **64**:327–36.

Weiss L (1985) *Principles of metastasis.* Academic Press Inc, New York.

Signalling mechanisms in cells

Alberts B (1998) The cell as a collection of protein machines: preparing the next generation of molecular biologists. *Cell*, **92**:291–4.

Huang S and Ingber DE (1999) The structural and mechanical complexity of cell growth control. *Nature Cell Biology*, **1**: 131–8.

Tjian R (1995) Molecular machines that control genes. *Scientific American*, **February**:38–45.

Inherited susceptibility to cancer

Crow JF (1999) The odds of losing at genetic roulette. *Nature*, **397**:293–4.

Eeles RA, Ponder BAJ, Easton DF, Horwich A, eds. (1996) *Genetic predisposition to cancer.* Chapman Hall Medical Publishers, London.

Lindor NM, Greene MH, Mayo Familial Cancer Programmme (1998) The concise handbook of family cancer syndromes. *J Natl Cancer Inst*, **90**:1039.

Tumour regression and protracted latency

Papac RJ (1996) Spontaneous regression of cancer. *Cancer Treatment Rev*, **22**:395–423.

Wheelock EF, Weinhold KJ, Levich J (1981) The tumor dormant state. *Adv Cancer Res*, **34**: 107–40.

Transfer of cancer cells between individuals

Ford AM, Ridge SA, Cabrera ME, Mahmoud H, Steel CM, Chan LC, *et al.* (1993) In utero rearrangements in the trithorax-related oncogene in infant leukaemias. *Nature*, **363**:358–60.

Hancock BW, Newlands ES, Berkowitz RS, eds. (1997) *Gestational trophoblastic disease.* Chapman & Hall Medical Publishers, London.

Holland E (1949) A case of transplacental metastasis of malignant melanoma from mother to foetus. *J Obstet Gynaecol*, **56**:529–36.

Penn I (1991) Donor transmitted disease: cancer. *Transpl Proc*, **23**:2629–31.

Scanlon EF, Hawkins RA, Fox WW, Smith WS (1965) Fatal homotransplanted melanoma. *Cancer*, **18**:782–9.

'Protective' inflammatory reactions and cancer

Balkwill F and Mantovani A (2001) Inflammation and cancer: back to Virchow? *Lancet*, **357**:539–45.

PART THREE

PARADOX OF PROGRESS: INDECENT EXPOSURES

Doctor Thomas sat over his dinner,
Though his wife was waiting to ring,
Rolling his bread into pellets;
Said, 'Cancer's a funny thing.

Nobody knows what the cause is,
Though some pretend they do;
It's like some hidden assassin
Waiting to strike at you.

Childless women get it,
And men when they retire;
It's as if there had to be some outlet
For their foiled creative fire.'

(From the poem 'Miss Gee' by W H Auden, 1937)

CHAPTER 13

IS CANCER AN EVOLUTIONARY INEVITABILITY?

U p until now, I've tried to provide an explanation of the evolutionary and biological mechanisms that underlie the development of a malignant clone of cells: an answer to the 'what is it?' question. It's time now to tackle the more difficult and broader issues of why and how. One way to look at the problem is as an extension of the mechanical view and to consider that cancer is solely a consequence of inherent design faults in a rather sophisticated machine. Even Rolls Royces can break down through no fault of the driver. There is an evolutionary argument for this as I suggested at the beginning of this book. Here it is again as a reprise. Cancer can be viewed as an inevitable consequence or intrinsic evolutionary penalty of two essential characteristics of successful complex organisms, including humans: first, the requirement for sustained proliferative or regenerative activity, survival tactics, and mobility in the tissue stem cells in long-lived animals, coupled with accessible lymphatic and vascular channels for migration; second, the evolutionary advantage of having genetic recombination or gene shuffling mechanisms coupled with a lack of complete fidelity in DNA copying and repair. Multiple physiological restraints have evolved via natural selection to accommodate or severely limit these lifetime risks but they can, and do, patently fail – under certain conditions. There are two circumstances in which failure might be expected.

In the beginning

The first few weeks and months after fertilization are a challenging time. It is during this period that waves of migrating stem cells and proliferation occur in the formation of our nervous system, muscle, kidneys, and so on. Even without the agency of mutagen exposure, damage to DNA may occur via the very active proliferation and oxidative metabolism of these cells. These molecular mishaps may then initiate *de novo* the process of cancer evolution in cells otherwise going about their normal embryonic or foetal business. It is not surprising either that it happens or that it is rare. Nature is imperfect but not that clumsy.

The majority of paediatric cancers are probably initiated in this critical prenatal period. Ask ten epidemiologists what 'causes' childhood cancer and I guarantee that you will get either a blank stare or ten different answers. The smarter ones amongst them will tell you that nobody knows. Which is true. But the usual assumption is still that 'something' causes it and for most epidemiologists, as for the public at large, the elusive 'something' is 'out there', cunningly avoiding detection. To be fair, it is excruciatingly difficult to design appropriate studies of childhood cancer aetiology given the rarity of the very many and various subtypes, but is the underlying premise correct? My guess, and it is just a guess, is that for at least some childhood cancers, there is no external causative agent. Their very low frequency would be compatible with the notion that the proximal cause of the mutations driving the emergence of a cancer clone is the inherent proliferative and oxidative stress of development itself, coupled with the imperfect fidelity of DNA management. In other words, an accident of nature – our internal nature, reflecting ancient biological rules, regulations, and, in this case, flaws. No different in principle than many of the 1 per cent congenital abnormalities that we see at birth in most human populations which are believed to reflect, in the most part, chance errors in the developmental programme driving a very complex task of structural engineering in the embryo.

If this were the case, then one would not expect the incidence rates of paediatric cancer to vary much, if at all, between different populations and over time. There is in fact some variation in recorded incidence rates but this could to some extent reflect accuracy of diagnoses and anyway it is, for most subtypes of cancer, only around two to threefold – of a very different magnitude from what is observed with typical adult cancers, as we will see later. One exception to this happens to be with the major type of childhood cancer – acute lymphoblastic leukaemia. For this, I believe there is another, paradoxical, explanation, but one very much in keeping with the theme of this book. This one you'll have to wait to hear about (or skip to the end of the book).

One would expect evolutionary adaptations to have minimized cancer risk during foetal and early life and indeed up to and including the reproductive period. It would not be possible to entirely prevent mutations and cancer occurring by endogenous mechanisms and chance, with or without any additional exogenous genotoxic exposure, but there should be some antique but successful trick up the adaptive sleeve to minimize the potential impact. And there is. The fail-safe device operational before birth is cell death and, as the ultimate sanction, spontaneous abortion. A substantial proportion of all conceptions are followed by foetal loss, many of which are unnoticed. If the evolutionary imperative is transmission of one's genes, then it might seem somewhat bizarre to have an inbuilt device to prevent this happening. On balance however, it may be tactically smarter to facilitate foetal loss rather than risk having offspring that are genetically damaged, might die when very young, or be at a disadvantage for later reproduction. Better to start again, especially for a species that puts so much energy into nurturing the unborn and newborn.

Recent research hints at how the default process might work. We're back on the p53 bus again. The function of p53 protein is activated following the sensing of the presence of DNA damage in cells and it then signals alternative options: either stop replicating DNA and repair the damage before proceeding, opt for a non-proliferative or quiescent status, or drop dead (the damaged cells that is). (Go back to page 62 if you've forgotten all this.) Molecular technology now allows us to ask the following question: what happens to developing mammalian foetuses if the gene making p53 protein is absent or inactive (in a so-called 'knock-out' mouse)? The answer surprised and disappointed biologists at first because essentially nothing happened. But the key follow-up question was – what happened if mice deprived of p53 protection were exposed before birth, whilst in the womb, to DNA-damaging irradiation? For normal mice with p53 intact, the exposure leads to a high rate of foetal losses by spontaneous abortion, plus a low rate of live births with congenital abnormalities. For the mice without p53, the converse was true; the majority of foetal mice were not aborted but were born with a variety of developmental abnormalities, and a high incidence of cancer in the following months (mostly leukaemia). The biological and evolutionary rationale here seems straight-forward enough. If p53, as a guardian of your genetic material, senses and signals DNA damage above a certain level beyond which repair processes are likely to be swamped, then the command is for cells to die. Up to a point, there is sufficient redundancy of cell number and function in the developing embryo that this loss can be accommodated. But, if substantial numbers of cells in an embryo or foetus die, then that embryo or foetus itself will not survive. It's brutal but, in evolutionary terms, it makes sense. Without the agency of p53 and cell death, there would probably be more children born with serious malformations and more cancer.

Of course cancer still does occur in young children, as do other congenital abnormalities. That these can slip through the p53 safety net is not surprising. Mutations initiating cancer clone emergence, if they are purely accidents of DNA replication, may not be detected by the p53 surveillance mechanism and if they occur relatively late in embryonic or foetal development, need not impede development to full term. The net result of these biological arrangements is that we finish up with a very low incidence rate of cancer in young children. The overall risk of any new born developing cancer up to the age of 15 years is around 1 in 800. Tragic though these cases are, the selective forces of evolution ignore or tolerate the low rate of biological error that produced these cancers. To stop all mutations, if it were possible, would be to stop evolution itself. To stop all clonal expansion would be to severely impede resilience and, downstream, reproductive success.

Towards the end

Survival into old age is one measure of human success and cancer looks like one price to pay. More than 60 years ago, A R Rich showed that over 25 per cent of men aged 70 years or more studied at autopsy had previously unrecognized invasive prostate carcinoma. The figure is higher still for men over 90. The average risk of a young man of 25 dying of cancer in the following five years is 50 times less than that of a man of 65. Clearly, cancer has got something to do with ageing and the most effective way to avoid it is to die young. But, other than statistical risk, what does it mean if we say that cancer is predominantly a disease of ageing individuals? One view is that cancer is an intrinsic part of the ageing process and for this possibility, we can find a biological rationale. Overall, around 80 per cent of cancers occur at an age that is post-reproductive for women and that should be so for men, or rather would be so in a more 'natural' environment. This suggests one possible mechanism for increased cancer risk. In post-reproductive older age, cell turnover in the renewable tissues continues relatively unabated. Oxidative stress in cells will extract an accumulative toll and spontaneous mutations should increase. A markedly increased level of genetic mishaps (ten to twentyfold) can be observed in blood cells and epithelial cells of old versus young individuals, though we have no way of knowing if these arise spontaneously or via some external insults. At the same time, we might expect the integrity of controls over both DNA management and clonal expansion to become less finely tuned or at least a little rusty with age. Along these lines, DNA repair capacity of cells from old rats is inferior to that of more youthful rodents and, in ageing humans, blood cell production appears to be monopolized by just a few semi-dominant clones. Given these signs of biological slippage, cancer might indeed be expected to increase as an inherent component of the ageing process.

Our programming as primate mammals has not anticipated or had time to adapt to our rapid acquisition of the ability to survive the rigours of post-reproductive life. There is no effective contingency plan for such a radical, though not unique, departure from the biological norm and it would be very surprising if it were otherwise. As the distinguished British biologists J B S Haldane and Peter Medawar both pointed out many years ago, the process of ageing in human beings lies beyond the influence of natural selection.[1] Our genetic heritage has to include instructions for stringent management and monitoring of DNA and clonal expansionist tendencies at the beginning of life. These processes should be sustainable for a lengthy period, and perhaps beyond their normal time frame of utility, but they might be expected to be blind to slippage towards the end.

One opinion on this view of cancer and ageing is that a key agency responsible for policing the problem loses interest or competence. MacFarlane Burnett, Australian doyen of the immune system, suggested that creeping senility of immunological surveillance held major responsibility for the excess of cancers in old age. But then he and some other immunologists, along with the distinguished American medical scientist and writer, Lewis Thomas, belonged to the club that believed a prime function and evolutionary rationale of the immune system was control of cancer. There has never, to my mind, been any cogent evidence for this view. One other, evolutionary, perspective on ageing involves an intriguing and plausible idea encapsulated by a less than handsome label – negative pleiotropy. The essence of this is that all the effort and energy expended on optimizing essential functions before and during reproductive life might incur a later penalty. This is the 'bad news' scenario since delayed penalties will actually be encouraged, indirectly, by natural selection. It's a dismal view on life but one very much in tune with the strident neo-Darwinian view that, biologically speaking, passing on one's genes is all that really counts. So, it all looks like bad tidings for oldies in the cancer stakes, doesn't it? But is it?

What would happen if, by accident or design, ageing was accelerated or slowed down? Would age-related cancer rates then be, correspondingly, increased or decreased? The nearest we can come to such an experiment is with Werner's syndrome. This is an exceedingly rare, genetically determined disorder of very premature ageing called progeria. Distressing symptoms occur before the age of 35 and include many we associate with ageing – greying hair and hair loss, cataracts, osteoporosis, skin wrinkling, and heart disease. There is also an increased incidence of tumours in comparison with young, age-matched controls. But these are principally of one kind – sarcoma – and most cases are non-malignant. There is no increase in carcinomas, the common cancer type that occurs at increasing frequency with age. Werner's syndrome may or may not be an appropriate parody of the ageing process but it provides little or no evidence that cancer is intrinsically linked to ageing itself. Some other things don't fit either. Tumours and cancers can be found in most animal species and in ageing animals held in captivity, but very few geriatric turtles and elephants die of cancer. Allegedly. Some reduced efficacy of DNA repair and of immune responses have been described in old cells and tissues but they are probably not of an order to account for cancer rates in old versus young people.

There are other very cogent reasons for suspecting that it takes more than intrinsic fallibility and a ticking clock to explain the likely incidence rates of cancer before this century and the currently very high rates of certain types of cancer in many societies. Take old age itself for starters. The average life span has changed dramatically over the past 10 000 years and particularly over the past 200 years, during which time it has roughly doubled in industrialized societies. Nevertheless, for many centuries there have been modest-sized cohorts of men and women who have lived well into their eighth or ninth decades. In earlier centuries, their eventual cause of death or any underlying internal cancer might have been missed, but from the eighteenth to early twentieth century this is highly unlikely to explain what appears to be a much lower incidence rate of cancer. By and large these Methuselah-like individuals didn't die of malignancy. In current Aborigine or hunter-gatherer societies, some individuals do live to be 70 to 90 years of age and estimates of age-associated cancer mortality in these groups are generally quite low or less than 10 per cent.

Other observations reveal, with some force, that old age and inherited or random errors in DNA cannot be the whole story for cancer. Why do the age-matched incidence rates of many adult cancers vary so dramatically (10 to 300-fold) between different parts of the world? We'll take a look later at the geography of cancer 'hot spots'. Why do some cancers have a socio-economic association both between and within countries (for example, cancers of the liver, stomach, lung, and oesophagus are biased towards the 'poor' end; prostate, breast, colon, melanoma, and childhood leukaemia towards the opposite pole of relative affluence)? Why do migrant populations appear to acquire the differential cancer risk of the host country? Why do urbanized black Africans develop the cancers of 'Western' societies (and other 'modern' diseases into the bargain)? And why have incidence rates been varying in the West – mostly up (melanoma, breast, non-Hodgkin's lymphoma, oesophageal cancer, pancreas) but some down (stomach) – in this century? Why do Mormon and Seventh Day Adventist men have lower rates of several types of cancer than other USA males? Presumably not divine intervention. There is little doubt what the answer to these striking variations in incidence is. Cancer rates and risks are primarily cultural variables.

Ageing then is a *correlate* not a *cause* of most cancers. The biological reason for this is that increased life span provides both the extended time frame within which there will be more opportunities for unrepaired or misrepaired DNA damage to be induced and to accumulate and the requisite protracted interval for a dominant clone to evolve and emerge. Armitage and Doll, intrigued by the exponential increase in cancer incidence with age, used mathematical modelling, in 1954 (long before our current genetic insights), to propose that the requirement for a succession of mutations (six or seven they calculated) might plausibly explain why living longer appears so risky as far as cancer is concerned. This was prescient and essentially correct, although the modelling failed to take into account successive waves of clonal expansion and selection. The running down of constraints and controls as we get older may have to take some responsibility for cancer but it's not the major player.

The conclusion to draw from these considerations is that minor clonal incursions or small tumours are inevitable and unavoidable in all of us. And at a much more modest level, malignant cancer may indeed be an inevitable and ubiquitous product of evolutionarily ancient design limitations. Don't ask me to put an accurate figure on it, but by modest I would guess a cumulative lifetime risk (that is, about 80 years) for cancer of somewhere around one to five per cent. But the bulk, some 90 per cent of cancers, are not inevitable. Their emergence requires assistance.

The social ratchet

There has been an enormous impact of lifestyle and changes in the structure and activities of society on cancer incidence rates. This view is endorsed by many leading epidemiologists whose studies have led to the commonly held view that some 90 per cent of cancers may have definable causes and be, in principle, preventable. These causes have been labelled as 'environmental' and this was rather loosely translated by some as pesticides and pollutant by-products of our petrochemical and nuclear industries. This view then sits ill at ease with the thesis by Peto, Doll, Cairns and others that lifestyle factors are the major causative factors. From which reverberates the riposte that attempting to pin the blame on lifestyle is akin to blaming the victim. And from these two different perspectives arises the inevitable conflict: is it society or the individual that is the main arbiter of risk? It's easy to see why this dualism takes on political overtones and engenders fierce advocacy.

I take the following view: for some 90 per cent of cancers, the major risk variables, other than constitutive genetics, are products, one way or another, of human social engineering over which any one of us exercises limited deliberate or informed choice in the normal course of events. By errors of commission or omission, we can be exposed to repeated or chronic toxic insults or sustained physiological stress to tissues. This can result in an increased frequency of mutations, either because the exposures involve substances that are directly DNA-damaging or because physiological stress translates to proliferative and oxidative stress to tissues and cells. Eventually DNA, like elastic, snaps. The process of chronic exposure and damage is wrapped up in important modulators of impact – our individual inherited genetics, eating habits, and energy balance. The former lottery, we can do little about; the latter two are very much social and cultural variables. Our rapid social evolution and exotic habits are badly out of line with our more pedestrian genetic legacy as naked apes. Not only do we live when we should naturally die or be eaten but we have altered our behaviour dramatically in ways which can very substantially increase risk. The net result is that over years and decades the risks of clonal escape increase proportionately. What else should one expect but more cancer, especially as we age? This is the social ratchet for cancer risk. But the ratchet is only effective because the biological base upon which it operates is intrinsically error-prone and equipped with cancerous credentials (for sound evolutionary reasons as we've seen) – a fatally discordant interplay of nature and nurture.

Of course many of our fellow travellers in the living world go in for remarkably bizarre lifestyles that ought to pose a threat to their well-being: the extremophiles (bacteria that can live close to 100°C or in virtually neat acid or alkali), dung-eating beetles, and poison-soaked frogs and snakes, for example. The difference is that they all represent the offspring of the first mutant survivor who learned to do the trick safely in the first place; they had their genetic passports correctly stamped. We are different – travelling the fast lane, socially speaking, but without genetic endorsement. Not that natural selection could, given infinite time, ever provide a genetic passport to a cancer-free society. Too much of the cancer burden occurs after our peak of reproductive activity.

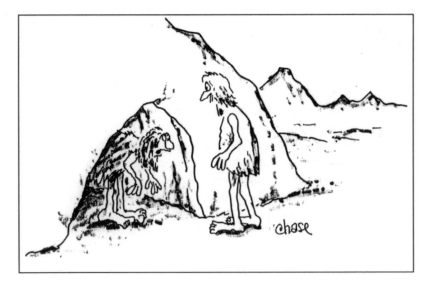

Figure 13.1 'I tried standing erect, but I kept banging my head!'

There is an impressive and informative, if complex, literature on human activities associated with cancer. This comes courtesy of epidemiological sleuths who have provided us with a formidable lexicon of clues to causality in cancer – and, no shortage of false trails. The less contentious components of this knowledge have entered the public domain and are beginning to influence educational, social, and commercial activities via persuasion or legislation. It is not the purpose of this book to catalogue all that has been discovered in this respect. Rather I wish to distil out those examples that may best illustrate the multiplicity of routes to cancer clone formation, the time frames involved, and the way in which human social attributes themselves change or evolve to challenge and provoke our genetic history and evolutionary legacy. To some extent, this will be a mirror on twentieth-century Westernized societies and lifestyles, but the social ratchet exacerbating cancer risks is much older, more widespread, and diverse than this. And it's perhaps in the broader context that we can best make sense of it all. If we are to make real inroads into the cancer toll, then the 'why?' question should be attributed at least equal status to the 'how?' question.

CHAPTER 14

AND THEN YOU SET FIRE TO IT?

To-bacco?
What's tobacco Walt?
It's a kind of leaf?
And you've bought eighty tonnes of it?
Let me get this straight Walt: you bought eighty tonnes of leaves?

This er, this may come of something of a surprise to you Walt
But come fall in England we're kind of up to our . . .

It isn't that kind of leaf?

What is it – a special food of some kind Walt?
Not exactly? It has a lot of different uses?
Like – what are some of its uses Walt?
Are you saying snuff, Walt?
What's snuff Walt?
You take a pinch of tobacco –
And shove it up your nose?
And it makes you sneeze eh?
I imagine it would Walt, ya.
Gee, the golden rod seems to do it pretty well already!
It has other uses though?
Yes, you can chew it?
Or put it in a pipe?
Or, you can shred it up and put it in a piece of paper and roll it up,
don't tell me Walt, don't tell me
– you stick it in your ear, right Walt?
Or between your lips?
Then what do you do to it Walt?

You set fire to it Walter?

(Imaginary conversation (by telephone) between Sir Walter Raleigh and Head of the West Indies Company in England)

(From Introducing tobacco to civilisation by Bob Newhart)

Whe'd's the greatest thing we have ever invented, our best trick: plant-ing corn, aeroplanes, Guinness? How about making a fire? Darwin gave this talent primacy over all but language acquisition as a crucial innovation in the development of humankind. The domesticated management of fire is a unique and universal human attribute. Fires are of course very much part of the natural world and have existed on the planet Earth as long as there has been combustible organics and, volcanically speaking, even before that. How man came to conquer such a magic and fearful element is the stuff of legends. Prometheus, the 'Bringer of Fire' in Ancient Greek mythology, stole it from Zeus and, for his pains, was chained to a rock whilst vultures nibbled daily at his liver. Sigmund Freud applied his vivid imagination to the problem. He suggested that 'primitive man was bound to regard fire as a symbol of the libido. The warmth that is radiated by fire calls up the same sensation that accompanies a state of sexual excitation, and the shape and movement of a flame suggest a phallus in activity.' But then mused Freud, there was a problem. Primitive man had an irresistible, sexually tinged urge to urinate on fire and overcoming this instinct was an essential step in man's mastery of the fiery element. Well, he would say that wouldn't he?

Exactly when our ancestors learnt the trick is a matter of vociferous debate amongst anthropologists. Some claim that the oldest evidence for deliberate or contained use of fire dates to over one million years ago with Australo-pithecines or *Homo erectus* in East Africa. Charcoal, burnt bones, ashes, and hearth-shaped structures have been attributed to the fiery activities of *Homo erectus* some half a million years ago in Choukoutien, south west of Beijing and in Terra Amata near Nice in the south of France, but the evidence is at best inconclusive and the conclusions contentious. Certainly by the late middle Pleistocene, some 150 000 to 200 000 years ago, Neanderthals and 'modern' *Homo sapiens* were constructing hearths and skilfully manipulating fire. How far back the talent stretches we simply don't know. Since some birds and mammals make use of natural fire to catch fleeing prey or enjoy partially burnt food, we can assume that opportunistic exploitation of fire, by say, en-couraging or containing it, preceded the development of skills for ignition, tendering, and domesticated use. How it was first mastered we can only guess. Legends of almost all native, indigenous, or Aborigine peoples provide a plethora of possibilities from the divine or baroque to the very plausible. But once one bright spark (so to speak) had it going, the rest, as Darwin himself suggested, was probably just mimicry. The talent for pyromania was either passed on or, most probably, independently acquired by tribal groups of *Homo sapiens*. Either way, we remain the only species whose members know how to light a fire.

Well, not quite. There is telling if anecdotal evidence that some of our nearest

Pongidae relatives, given a little prompting, can express some of the skills required. Bongo, a beer-swilling chimpanzee in Johannesburg Zoo, was taught by his former keeper how to light a cigarette. He not only became addicted to the pleasure but taught himself how to light a new cigarette up from the dying embers of the previous one. Another chimp, in an adjacent cage, acquired, by mimicry alone, the same remarkable ability. So the physical dexterity was there; what was needed was real incentive and social contacts to facilitate mimicry.

Whoever deserves the credit for making the first fire, and whenever, Darwin was surely correct in regarding this as a very smart move in evolutionary terms. One of our best. We could keep warm in inclement climates, facilitating survival and migration from the tropics. We could inhabit dark caves, and after a while, learn how to decorate their walls. We became culinary wizards, cooking and then eating otherwise unpalatable, indigestible, infectious, or poisonous food.[2] And then we could scare off potential predators. One can imagine that sitting around a fire benefited social cohesion and the elaboration of language. Smoke from fires provided the first deliberate or inadvertent long-distance signals of human presence in a territory. Even isolated human groups that have failed to invent the wheel know that fire is a good idea, though Jared Diamond tells that Tasmanian Aborigines apparently forgot how to do it for a while. The Jarawa aboriginal inhabitants of the Adaman Islands in the Bay of Bengal are perhaps the only living peoples who have yet to work it out.

But fire and smoke have a downside. First, they can burn your skin and your house or choke you to death and, second, the natural or carboniferous materials that are used generate not only heat but invisible and poisonous products of combustion. In this respect, lighting fires, in one form or another, has been the longest-running uncontrolled human experiment in chemistry. Natural fuel sources – coal, shale, oil, and living (or dead) organisms have an extraordinarily complex chemical composition. When these substances are fired, their atoms shake and chemistry changes. New molecules are generated, by pyrolysis, and accumulate as products of partial combustion in residue tars and, to some extent, in smoke. Tobacco tar, for example, is a cocktail of baroque complexity: over 5000 substances of which 40 or more are potentially carcinogenic. You might imagine that our evolutionary history will not have prepared our skin, mouth, airways, gut, and their constituent cells and genes, for persistent and fiery chemical abuse. The good news is that we are quite well endowed with detoxification mechanisms in cells that can neutralize almost all of the potential carcinogens in tar, smoke, and oil. Most of these chemicals do exist in the natural world at low level, either synthesized by plants or as products of natural combustion as in forest fires or peat formation. The bad news is that these metabolic processes can be outpaced or satiated by excessive or chronic exposure, and, paradoxically, actually activate DNA-damaging or carcinogenic chemicals as transient intermediates in a detoxification pathway. Cancer is then one consequence of chronic or excessive exposure to products of carboniferous combustion – different types of cancer in different tissues, depending upon the route of exposure.

The great weed

> Hun-Hunahpú and Vucab-Hunahpú entered the House of Gloom. There they were given their fat-pine sticks, a single lighted stick ... together with a lighted cigar for each of them which the lords had sent.
>
> *(From The Popol Vuh, the sacred book of the ancient Quiché Maya)*

Of all the cancers, tobacco-associated oral and lung cancers are the ones which most unequivocally reflect a conflict between biological evolution and the social ratchet of pleasurable behaviour and commercial gain. The case for cigarette smoking and lung cancer has been so well exposed and generally accepted in most developed countries that it hardly needs reiteration here. However, the historical and cultural context in which the twentieth-century epidemic of lung cancer developed is fascinating in its own right and in many ways a mirror on human, and particular European or Western culture. This perspective may help us to understand better the broader context and meaning of the word 'cause' as applied to cancer – and how our inherent biology can be subjected to social and commercial strangulation. We are also much better placed now to interrelate patterns of smoking and chemistry of tar with the underlying evolutionary biology of cancer cells.

Christopher Columbus and his fellow voyagers were the first Europeans, in 1492, to see native Indians indulging in what seemed to them the extraordinary habit of smoking – inhaling the smoke of grasses via tube-shaped plant leaves called tobaccos. What Columbus observed was novel for him but for native American Indians, this was a cultural habit that can be traced back for centuries and perhaps to as long ago as 2500 BC.

The pleasurable, narcotic, and medicinal properties of inhaled smoke have a very long historical pedigree that has pervaded most human cultures. Throw a few sweet or aromatic herbs and other plants on the fire and there you have it. Fiery incense or perfumed smoke has been an ancient offering to the gods by priests and shamans from ancient Egypt and Mesopotamia to the Mayans of central America. Both Greeks and Romans believed in medicinal benefits of inhaling smoke from burning plants (laurel or coltsfoot for example). Pliny recommended drawing in the smoke through a reed (that is, smoking) for obstinate coughs. Mayan priests are pictured on temple reliefs in the Yucatan peninsula blowing smoke from a tube and were perhaps the first to smoke in the sense we recognize today, using rolled-up palm leaves, reeds, or bamboo as a tube to hold powdered leaves. At his royal investiture, the Aztec king Moctezuma was said to have had placed around his neck a small gourd in which to keep tobacco – 'which is strength for the road'. And it was the tobacco plant, a rampant weed, that the Mayan, Aztec, and other indigenous Indians of Central America, Mexico, and the Antilles Islands had unique access to.

Many different plants and herbs were used for burning incense or smoking but one wild and abundant species held special appeal for its rich narcotic properties. Its Latin name, *Nicotiana tabacum*, was attributed as an accolade to Jean Nicot, the fifteenth-century French Ambassador to Lisbon and advocate for its use amongst the affluent and powerful in France and the rest of Western Europe. By the time the Spanish soldiers and adventurers were introduced to tobacco in the Caribbean, the habit of smoking was culturally entrenched throughout Central America, into Brazil and Venezuela, and north into the eastern United States and Canada where elaborate pipes, the red clay calumet, and ritual smoking were an integral part of social life. Spanish seamen took up the habit and, along with fellow seafarers from Portugal, England, and the Netherlands, played a major role in disseminating the smoking weed around the world. From the seventeenth-century Thirty Years' War to the Napoleonic campaigns, the Crimean War (1865), and, most spectacularly, the First World War, smoking by soldiers was encouraged by their commanders. Perhaps for good reason – tobacco's narcotic properties could nullify both fear and hunger. The end result? Fields full of the dead or addicted.

For health and wealth?

Smoking was not simply an acquired habit. The reasons for its successful penetration into all levels of European society had multiple causes, including its supposed medicinal benefits and its undoubted revenue benefits. Tobacco was considered almost as a universal panacea with therapeutic virtues for a variety of afflictions, including toothache, infections, skin problems, wounds, burns, dropsy, piles, gout, headaches, deafness, and, believe it or not, cancer. So read the instructions carefully:

> The drie leaves are used to taken in a pipe set on fire and suckt into the stomache, and thrust forth againe at the nostrils the parts of the head.

> (J Gerard, 1597)

And then, by the same writer:

> Some use to drink it (as is termed for inhaled smoke) for wantonnese or rather custome, and cannot forleave it, no, not in the midst of their dinner, which kind of taking is unwholesome and dangerous.

More especially, tobacco smoke was considered to be a disinfectant and to protect against the plague. Doctors had little to offer in the face of the intermittent plagues and pestilence that rampaged through Europe in the seventeenth and eighteenth centuries. Cursory observations and anecdotes hinted that those who smoked might be protected and doctors promulgated the idea of smoking as a prophylactic. Irresistible wasn't it? Even the boys at England's premier private school (Eton) were compelled to smoke first thing in the morning as a disinfective procedure. Protection against contagion was a godsend. Dr Johannes Neader of Bremen was one of tobacco's greatest apologists. His medical treatise of 1622, extolling the virtues of the great weed, was sent to doctors throughout Europe and included the claim that smoking it offered protection against the great pox (Syphilis). The pox, along with tobacco itself and the potato, was one of the supreme gifts of the conquered New World to the old. However, as Dr Wilhelm van der Meer observed, whilst tobacco might be good for a cold in the head, the evidence for any efficacy against the pox was at best unconvincing and a man might be better advised to avoid brothels. Dr van der Meer had a balanced view of the problem. He also chastized the church for its opinion that tobacco was evil because of its barbarian origins. By this criteria, he argued, some thousands of plants, including the eternal rhubarb, would have to be rejected.

Within 50 years of tobacco's introduction to Europe, many governments levied duty or taxes on importation and sales. Competition between national rivals for export from the New World countries sparked trade wars and high-seas piracy. New York probably owes its English name, rather than its former Dutch title, to arguments between the Virginian English and Dutch New Amsterdamers over tobacco trade and smuggling. Eventually governments throughout Europe were forced to take a more systematic approach to control with monopolies based either on a private concession (as first adopted in Venice), purchased by affluent merchants, or central government control.

Tobacco was an ace bargaining card in international trade with the huge sums of money at stake matching the political consequences in some cases. William Penn is said to have negotiated, over a smoking conference, the purchase of the territory that is now the State of Pennsylvania from the indigenous Indians for a deal that included 300 pipes, 100 baskets of tobacco, 20 snuffboxes, and 100 jew's harps. Benjamin Franklin financed the war of independence against the British in some considerable measure (two million French louis) by providing the French 'fermiers généraux' with Virginian tobacco. There was therefore nothing new about the insatiable greed of twentieth-century governments and companies for revenue riches from tobacco; only the degree of it.

Advocates and critics

Europe with its smoking taverns (tabagies in England) underwent changes in tobacco fashion as Dutch clay pipes for the masses, snuff for the nobs, and, in the seventeenth century, cigars from Cuba and cigarettes from Brazil waxed and waned in popularity. From the sixteenth through to the nineteenth century, there were both prominent and vocal critics and advocates for tobacco. Emperors, kings, popes, philosophers, and poets railed against the habit, but their sentiments or edicts were either ignored or overturned. Peter the Great (seventeenth-century Czar of Russia) on the other hand was a great fan of smoking (as well as most other hedonistic pursuits). Goethe and Napoleon hated smoking, as did Queen Victoria. Turkish poets on the other hand regarded tobacco as one of the four cushions of the divan of delight along with opium, coffee, and wine. But for one infamous Ottoman, Sultan Murad the Cruel, smoking was a foul sin punishable by death. The last emperor of the Ming dynasty, Tsung Cheng, issued an edict against smoking in 1641 but the Manchus who conquered Peking after the revolution in 1644 were inveterate smokers and paved the way for China to lead the way, as they do still today, in the use of the respiratory passages as living chimneys.

Sir Walter Raleigh is credited with the import into England of the tobacco plant (as now immortalized in Bob Newhart's hilarious skit *And then you set fire to it Walt?*). Sir Walter of course lost his head, some say whilst enjoying his last smoke. He was executed on the orders of King James I who wasn't too enamoured with tobacco either. One year after succession to the English throne he published, anonymously, his diatribe *A counter-blaste to tobacco* (1604). Scottish Jimmy was not a man to mince his words:

> For Tobacco being a common herbe, which (though under divers names) growes almost everywhere, was first found out by some of the barbarous Indians, to be a Preservative, or Antidot against the Pockes, a filthy disease, whereunto these barbarous people are (as all men know) very much subject, what through the uncleanly and adust constitution of their bodies, and what through the intemperate heate of their Climate: so that as from them was first brought into Christendome, that most detestable disease, so from them likewise was first brought this use of Tobacco, as a stinking and unsavorie Antidot, for so corrupted and execrable a Maladie, the stinking Suffumigation whereof they yet use against that disease, making so one canker or venime to eate out another.

and

> A custome lothsome to the eye, hateful to the Nose, harmeful to the braine, dangerous to the Lungs, and the blacke, stinking fume thereof, neerest resembling the horrible Stigian smoke of the pit that is bottomelesse.

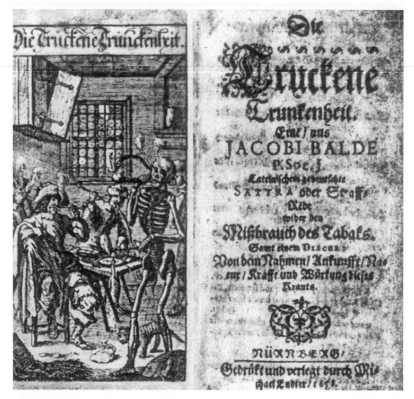

Figure 14.1 Title and frontpiece to Jakob Blade's satire on the abuse of tobacco *Die truckene trunkenheit* (Drunk without drinking), 1658; and a quote from the same Jesuit priest, 'What difference is there between a smoker and a suicide, except one takes longer to kill himself than the other?'

From time to time, prohibition has been temporarily imposed – in the city of Cologne, in the streets of Berlin, in St Peter's church in Rome. Usually these bans reflected the very real concerns of fire risk. In more recent times, 12 states of the USA banned tobacco smoking as did Hitler and the National Socialist Party in Nazi Germany. But this crude tactic, as other examples testify, is seldom effective when narcotic rewards, human pleasure, and monetary gain are at stake.

The cancerous kick

The link with cancer didn't pass unobserved either. In 1761 in London, John Hill – doctor, botanist, playwright, and polymath – published a one-shilling pamphlet cautioning against the immoderate use of tobacco snuff. He described several cases of fatal polypuses of the nose or nasal carcinoma in men who were heavy, long-term users of snuff and he proferred the following advice: 'no man should venture upon snuff, who is not sure that he is not so far liable to cancer: and no man can be sure of that.' This was one of the first epidemiological links for cancer and was followed by observations of Samuel Thomas von Soemmering in 1795 on pipe smoking and cancer of the lip. Over the next hundred years, pipe smoking became more widely recognized as being associated with oral cancer and especially cancer of the lower lip and tongue. When Yankee General and ex-President Ulysses S Grant died of throat cancer in 1885, his doctors concluded that his long-standing predilection to cigars was the likely cause.

As fashions of tobacco use have changed, so too have the patterns of cancer risk. What matters here are the dose and delivery form of the tobacco combustibles and inhalation practice. These collectively determine what tissue is most subjected to persistent carcinogenic challenge. For snuff, the nose is the obvious hot spot. For pipe smoking and tobacco chewing, the oral cavity is the prime target (including lips and tongue, as well as the throat) as it is for certain cigarettes, for example many French makes, whose alkaline nature ensures more effective absorption in the oral surfaces making inhalation less necessary for a nicotine kick. At the beginning of the twentieth century, an American clinician, Dr R Abbe, provided compelling evidence that oral cancer was linked to tobacco exposure. All but one of his 90 patients were avid consumers of the great weed. His evidence was in part anecdotal, but instructive nonetheless: a patient presented with one of the most virulent cancers of the tongue he had ever seen. Abbe asked her how it all began: 'I have, all my life, taken a small toothbrush in my right hand, dipped it in snuff and rubbed it hard on my tongue.'

The oral cavity is also the hot spot for cancers associated with some of the more exotic smoking styles developed in India and other parts of South East Asia. These include the bidi and the chutta. The bidi is made from dried temburni leaf stuffed with tobacco – less tobacco and less smoke than conventional cigarettes but, for the millions who continue to enjoy it, more tar, more carcinogens, and more nicotine. Chutta is made with rolled tobacco leaf and in some parts of India is used by women in a rather bizarre fashion that Bob Newhart would appreciate (with the lighted end inside the mouth - see Fig. 14.2). A consequence of this predilection for these fire-eating females is a high incidence of cancers of the palate. In South East Asia also, non-incinerated or smokeless tobacco has been consumed for centuries. It is estimated that over 200 million people currently chew betel quid (colloquially known as pan) which is a mixture of the betel leaf, areca nut, slaked lime, and, usually, tobacco. The tobacco can be in the form of a gel mixed with herbs and

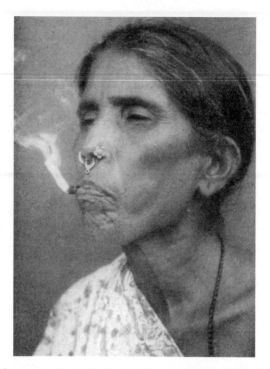

Figure 14.2 Indian women in Andhra Pradesh have acquired the habit of smoking chutta cigars with the burning end inside the mouth.

spices (kivam) or flaked with spices (zardu). Those that include the tobacco ingredient are at high risk of oral cancer, especially if they retain the quid in their mouths for some hours (long enough for the alkaline condition to facilitate release of tobacco carcinogens without the agency of fire). Chromosome abnormalities can be detected in the buccal epithelial cells of healthy quid chewers to an extent that parallels the duration of chewing and the number of quids used per day: a silent clock ticking. Lethal lesions of the oral cavity are described in Indian medical texts from around 600 BC. Since chewing betel quid also backtracks to this period or beyond, it is likely that oral cancers associated with this social custom have a very long track record indeed.

For pipe smokers, the lower lip appears to be more at risk than the upper, and it may be that the damage elicited by heat exacerbates the impact of tobacco carcinogens. For the traditional high tar cigarette, and particularly with inhalation, the major bronchial tracts incur the highest insult and consequent cancer rate (squamous bronchial carcinoma).

In the first half of the twentieth century, lung cancer, formerly considered to be a very rare disease, began to be increasingly diagnosed and many doctors and scientists both in the USA and Europe, and particularly in Nazi Germany, voiced their suspicion that cigarette smoking might be the cause. But it took until 1950 for epidemiologists, Doll and Hill in the UK, and Wynder and Graham in the USA, to provide persuasive epidemiological evidence for the strong association between tobacco smoking and lung cancer risk. By then, and following two world wars, smoking of mass-produced and relatively cheap cigarettes was culturally entrenched and the twentieth-century epidemic of lung cancer was well established.

Even after the landmark epidemiological studies, there were vocal sceptics including not only tobacco lobbyists with vested interests but academics as well. As Doll and Hill acknowledged at the time, correlation doesn't necessarily mean or prove causality. Animal experiments were not very helpful; it isn't immediately obvious how one would persuade laboratory rodents to mimic human smoking. Various smoke propelling gadgets were used, but with little impact. There are a number of reasons why these experiments failed to deliver a clear verdict, not least that rodents, being evolutionarily adapted to living near the ground, have nasal trabeculae that can filter out potentially noxious pulmonary contaminants. For us upright creatures, it's been pretty much free passage.

But could there be other non-causal explanations of the link between smoking and cancer? Some thought so. Sir Ronald Fisher, the distinguished British statistician and geneticist, launched something of a mini-crusade against the medical establishment for what he regarded as uncritical acceptance of proof of causality that unreasonably condemned what he regarded as the 'mild and soothing weed'. Wasn't it equally or more likely, he argued, that the tendency to smoke cigarettes and develop lung cancer were separate attributes of some common genetic, inherited factor? He conjured up some evidence from studies of twins that smoking preferences might be subject to genetic control but seemed blind to the fact that lung cancer had escalated in the first half of the twentieth century and that risk increased in proportion to the number of cigarettes consumed. Still, for some, Fisher's argument was attractive, especially for those who believed everything in human behaviour could be reduced to inviolate genetics. None more so than Hans Eysenck, the London-based psychologist. Papers and a book were published purporting to support the Fisher fallacy by demonstrating that cigarette smokers were a particular genetic breed: stocky, sanguine extroverts. Here we are back with the ghost of Galen reprising the myth of the cancer personality. That this crazy behavioural correlation could be given equal causal merit with chemical carcinogenesis was, even in the 1960s, a vivid illustration of how naïve intelligent men can be.

That it took so long to recognize a causal coupling between tobacco smoking and death and even longer to take any effective action has been disastrous. In part, the fatal delay reflects the lack of epidemiological expertise prior to the late 1940s. Undoubtedly the long interval of two to five decades between taking up smoking and paying the price, plus the fact that not all smokers die of lung cancer (see box on page 135), provided some disguise of the causal link and real risk. We now understand from the biology of cancer why such a long interval or latency is to be expected and why not all those exposed will develop cancer in the time available or before something else kills them. The necessary sequential accumulation of mutations in an evolving cancer clone also explains the observation that even for long-time smokers, giving up can lower the risk of lung cancer emerging. The persistent and long-term barrage of DNA-damaging chemicals in tar and smoke is the generator that makes the Darwinian evolution of cancer more likely to happen and pharmacological addiction to nicotine is the oil that lubricates the engine. But then ignorance of mechanism isn't an excuse is it?

The pusher's pursuit of profit

The magnitude of this twentieth-century epidemic of tobacco-related death is mind boggling. The International Agency for Research on Cancer, eminent epidemiologists including Richard Peto, the USA Surgeon General's office, and others have calculated the number of deaths attributable to cigarette smoking worldwide and provided indications of what is still too come. Currently between two and four million adults a year die of smoking-related diseases or, as Richard Peto more bluntly puts it, are killed by tobacco. Some 40 per cent of these have lung cancers. Other causes of death include cancers of the mouth, pharynx, and larynx, ischaemic heart disease, aortic aneurysms, and obstructive lung diseases. In fact, this list is longer as at least 30 conditions that are life-threatening, chronic, or debilitating are either directly linked to tobacco exposure or exacerbated by smoking. Cigarette smoking also increases the risk of cancers of the pancreas, kidney, and bladder – presumably by carcinogens entering the bloodstream.

Cigarette smoking is declining in some developed countries but the benefits in terms of lowered incidence of lung cancer are not as great as might have been anticipated and an awful paradox is emerging. Cancers of the lung bronchi (squamous cell carcinomas) are decreasing but the previously rare adeno-carcinomas of the lung are increasing substantially amongst smokers, and especially in women. These tumours arise from the deeper branch ends of the lung tree (the alveoli), and the most plausible explanation for their startling increase is that smokers have adopted the habit of inhaling more deeply to obtain their nicotine fix from their 'milder' cigarettes. Cigarettes are just bad news.

Cigarettes, lies, and videotape

Dr Wakeman: You must be trying to get me to admit that smoking is harmful. Apple sauce is harmful if you get too much of it.

Questioner: I don't think many people are dying of apple sauce.

Dr Wakeman: They're not eating that much. I think that if the company as a whole believed cigarettes were really harmful, we would be out of business. We're a very moralistic company.

(Dr Wakeman, Vice President of Phillip Morris, questioned in 'Death in the West', Thames TV, 1976)

In the USA, after years of cover up and prevarication, the major companies involved in the biggest health scandal of the twentieth century are finally showing signs of coming out in the open on the risk attributable to their product – coming out or being reluctantly extradited. The consequences are substantial in terms of likely regulation of a now recognized addictive drug (nicotine in tobacco) and recovery of medical costs. The long latency of lung cancer due to smoking may have helped disguise this lethal connection for the first half of the twentieth-century, allowing the profiteers a veil of innocence, but it beggars belief that as recently as 1994 Chief Executives of seven major cigarette manufacturers could testify under oath before the USA Government House Health and Environment Committee that they did not believe that nicotine was addictive or that cigarette smoking caused lung cancer. Whether this view was the genuine product of a bizarre collective logic, pathetic ignorance, or a downright lie, we will only know for sure when one of the executives spills the beans in his, no doubt lucrative, memoirs. But we can guess the answer. The Brown and Williamson documents leaked from one major cigarette manufacturer and now available on the internet provide graphic evidence that the tobacco trade have known for many years that their product was an addictive killer.

In China, India, eastern Europe, and Africa, the story is very different with dangerous trends in the opposite direction accelerating as the tobacco giants reset their targets in a global market. It would be comically amusing, if it wasn't so murderously tragic, that there are cigarettes marketed in Africa called 'Life' and another brand more appropriately labelled as 'Death'. One third of the world's smokers are Chinese. The majority of Chinese men smoke, including many doctors. Although their government show encouraging signs of respond- ing to the epidemic that threatens to overwhelm them, it is economically shackled: tobacco is their largest industrial source of tax revenue (equivalent to some ten billion USA dollars in 1996 alone). On current estimates, including recent studies in China itself, Oxford-based Peto and his colleagues calculate that one third of young Chinese men smoking now will die of a tobacco-related illness during the first half of the twenty-first century providing an accumulative death toll of around 100 million. On a worldwide scale, Peto calculates that, based on current trends, the annual death rate will increase to 10 million a year by 2030 and half of these individuals will be only 35 to 70 years of age. It's an absolute bloody disaster; a monumental obscenity.

In one very real sense the major cause of lung cancer has been unequivocally established as DNA-damaging chemical carcinogens in the combustion products of the inhaled tar and smoke. Inhalation, as President Clinton acknowledged in another context, is what counts. Cigarette smoke and particularly residue tars contain an extraordinary chemical mix, including several thousand substances of which over 40 can damage DNA and are demonstrably carcinogenic to rodent skin. The most potent of these are benzo(a)pyrene and nitrosamines. Chemical footprints of these lethal molecules can be detected attached to DNA in the lungs of smokers and in amounts that parallel their smoking habits. Experimentally, adducts or products of metabolized benzo(a)-pyrene, one of the most potent carcinogens in tobacco tar, have been shown to physically associate with selective regions of the *p53* gene which constitute the hot spots for mutation in lung cancers. This degree of genetic targeting by a carcinogen is somewhat surprising; we have tended to regard such offensive molecules as rather indiscriminate in their damage. Be that as it may, this evidence is highly incriminating. Other chromosomal or molecular abnormalities characteristic of lung cancer cells can be detected in the bronchial washing of individuals who do not (yet) have cancer – and at a level that parallels their cumulative smoking experience. A smoking gun if ever there was one. How much more evidence do you want?

The molecular biology and epidemiology together provide incontrovertible evidence, though for any individual smoking victim there can never be complete certainty that smoking caused his or her death. Except in the case of two doctors as noted by Sir Richard Doll in his remarkable 40-year survey of mortality causes and smoking habits in UK doctors. These two both died as a result of a fire caused by smoking in bed. The same fate almost befell General de Gaulle, who, like many of his French compatriots, was an ardent cigarette smoker. He gave up the habit after setting fire to his bed.

There is a somewhat different perspective on cancer causation. Harvard biologist, Richard Lewontin and Robert Proctor, science historian at Penn State University, have both argued persuasively that 'cause' should be considered in a broader context than those proximal events or agents, such as carcinogens in cigarette tar, that trigger disease and should include social, commercial, and political factors that have tangibly influenced risk. The whole social and commercial history of tobacco use outside of its original indigenous Indian context is, in a way, part of the route to chaos. In this sense also, the twentieth-century lung cancer epidemic was hugely facilitated by the invention of cigarette-making machines in the 1880s, the wholesale provision of free cigarettes to hundreds of thousands of soldiers in two world wars (creating armies addicted to the invisible pull of nicotine), the commercialization of production and sales much of which has been in callous disregard of recognized lethal consequences, and last, but not least, politicians whose thirst for tax revenue, sponsorship, or votes put them in bed with the tobacco lobby. It's a shoddy and tragic but very human tale of ignorance, culpability, and greed. Fire was and still is a great idea. Smoking plant leaves has had undoubted positive benefits too. Would J S Bach, Mark Twain, Evelyn Waugh, and other artistic thoroughbreds who were addicts have been so creative without it? Who knows?

(Un)Lucky strike?

There is a mystery here – I don't think even Professor Doll could elucidate it – the mystery of the thousands of people who had smoked like chimneys without coming to any harm.

(The journalist, Bernard Levin, 1997)

Tobacco's residual tar may be only drip-fed to the bronchial linings via cigarette smoking but the cumulative burden of toxic junk is remarkable. The lungs of a 'pack a day' man smoking for 40 years will have been the repository for 7 to 8 kilograms of tar. Even under these circumstances, not all ageing and long-term smokers will develop lung cancer to the point of a clinical diagnosis. Around one in ten of those who smoke 15 to 25 cigarettes a day will have lung cancer by age 75 years. Heavy smokers (more than 25 a day) suffer this fate at a higher rate still. Some will still escape this penalty but for reasons that call for no celebration – they are dying from other smoking-related causes. Additionally, for every 20 lung cancer patients in the USA or Europe who smoke, there will be, on average, one non-smoker with a similar diagnosis. That lung cancer can occasionally arise by other routes is not at all at odds with cigarette smoking being the major causal route to trouble: exclusivity in cancer causation is neither assumed nor required.

But the fact that even for long-time smokers, only a minority do develop lung cancer does beg an obvious question: assuming all the smokers in any cohort have the same history in terms of when they started, total years' worth of consumption, and tar yields of the brands they puffed, what's so special about the one with cancer versus the other nine without? He is of course, by definition, a different and unique individual, with his own genetic prescription for variation – and this might have loaded the dice against him. However, in contrast to the situation with cancers of the breast, colon, and prostate, there is no evidence for inherited mutant genes that can explain the occurrence of lung cancer. But other inherited genes could have made a difference. Potentially carcinogenic chemicals can be detoxified by cells but, paradoxically, activated as an intermediary step in this process. These activities are executed by enzymes and, as an outbred species, we vary significantly in how proficient our enzymes are. This variation in turn is prescribed by a natural sequence diversity (or alleles) in the individual inherited genes involved. The luck of the parental draw determines that those individuals who develop lung cancer and smoke heavily are, on average, somewhat more likely than equivalent smokers who escape to have the genotype that enhances carcinogen activity of benzo(a)pyrene, nitro-samines, and other DNA-damaging chemicals in tobacco tar and smoke. The relative risk is around twofold. In this respect, the oldest woman in western Europe (Madame Jeanne Calment) who died, but not of cancer, at 122 years of age, can perhaps thank her parents for escaping the penalty of a lifelong habit of smoking. Likewise others: '*If I'd taken my doctor's advice and quit smoking when he advised me to, I wouldn't have lived to go to his funeral.*' (George Burns at 98 years of age and still smoking 10 cigars a day.)

But the handicap or bonus of the parental draw is insufficient to explain the one in ten score. Studies comparing identical and non-identical twins, with essentially the same smoking history within each pair, have been revealing. They indicate that identical twins do not have a higher rate of concordance for lung cancer than non-identical twins – that is, no greater chance of both having lung cancer, despite the same carcinogen barrage. In most cases, only one of the twin pair developed lung cancer. The conclusion to draw is that whilst neither twin would be likely to have had lung cancer without smoking, it was in the end luck that tipped the balance and determined who did and who did not. And by luck here I mean the lottery of which genes in which cells incurred critical hits or a full set of hits; in other words, the bad luck of the (un)lucky strikes, when and how often during 50 years of risk taking.

So, just suppose we could rewind the life tape of 100 aged men that had smoked 15 to 25 cigarettes a day all their adult lives, including 10 that developed lung cancer, and another 100 that were cancer-free non-smokers. And then we gave them all the opportunity to do it all again. What would be the outcome of this parable? If we found that the same 10 individuals developed lung cancer, we would either have to revisit the role of inherited genetics in lung cancer or perhaps take a closer look at their other personal idiosyncrasies, in diet for example. That diets can provide some modest protection against lung cancer is clear and some smokers are impoverished in this respect. But my guess is that on the rerun there would again be around 10 cases of lung cancer and that all 10 would be in the smoking brigade but most, or possibly all, would be a different 10 men from those with lung cancer in the first run. All the smokers will have had genetic damage in their bronchial epithelium and many would have had some mini-cancers (detectable by current 'smart' techniques) but, as with the discordant identical twins, it will have been chance, luck, or bad luck, that finally tipped the balance – that pushed the clonal evolution of cancer cells to the point of no return.

And then if, in our imaginary reprise, we could run the tape longer than before, miraculously staving off death from other causes (including those that are linked to tobacco consumption), what would happen? It is highly likely that considerably more than 10 per cent of those continuing to smoke would develop lung cancer. Eventually, given enough time, most or all of the puffing runners would surely succumb. Any survivors would be fortunate indeed – and very interesting.

Of course I don't know this to be true; it's just a fantasy – the same one that can be applied to other outcomes that are the product of cumulative evolutionary accidents. Stephen Jay Gould has championed the view that if we could wind back the whole of life's tape for 500 million years, then the rerun would produce a very different outcome in terms of species diversity, winners, and losers. And we probably wouldn't be here to confirm the success of the prediction.

Don't be confused here; cigarette smoking is by some distance the major determinant of lung cancer risk and the more anyone smokes, and the longer they smoke, then the greater the risk. But we need to paint with a broader brush to see the full picture; like a complicated tapestry, if you stand too close, the picture gets blurred.

Heat in the kitchen

Our lungs can also be exposed to other inhaled insults from smoking fires that induce mutations and cancer, with or without an additive risk from cigarette smoking. One striking example concerns China. During the 1970s, Xuan Wei county in southern China had one of the highest rates of lung cancer in the whole of China. What was odd about this was that the mortality rate for women was as high as that of men, despite the fact that less than 0.1 per cent of women smoked cigarettes, compared with almost 50 per cent of the men.

Comparison of widely different rates of lung cancer between different communes within the province revealed that the explanation was almost certainly the burning indoors of smoky coal, as opposed to smokeless coal or wood, during the winter months, and the inhalation of the complex organic products of this combustion. The same domestic explanation is believed to apply to a tenfold variation in lung cancer rates of non-smokers in different cities in China.

There are a few other instances where the male predominance of lung cancer is broken. Maori women have long suffered from high rates of lung cancer but for them it is no mystery. The cultural mores of the Maoris were such that there was no prejudice against women taking up the weed when it was first introduced by Europeans. Chinese women in Shanghai, Hong Kong, Singapore, and the USA have a remarkably high rate of a form of cancer that has not been traditionally associated with smoking – lung adenocarcinoma. Although there is now a link between this type of cancer and deeper inhalation of low-tar, low-nicotine cigarettes, the great majority of these Chinese women do not smoke at all. Epidemiological evidence suggests that the explanation may be persistent and excess inhalation of hot cooking oil vapours, particularly from stir-frying and deep frying in sesame, peanut, rape-seed, and other volatile oils.

Women in other traditional societies may have suffered a similar fate. Prior to the 1960s, the few cases of lung cancer in Inuits living in the Canadian Arctic were in females. This was before cigarette smoking became prevalent in their society and has been plausibly suggested to be linked with the women's exclusive role in the home of tending lamps fuelled by seal oils. These emit very sooty smoke to which the women would have been persistently exposed within their small, confined living spaces. We can assume that such exposures and possibly such consequences have been a long-running saga since settlement in these Arctic wastelands some 15 000 to 25 000 years ago. In this respect, the Mummies of Qilakitsoq were revealing. These are the well-preserved bodies of one infant, one child, and six adult women found at a burial site in Western Greenland in 1972; dating places their deaths at around 1475, give or take 50 years. Their bodies, clothes, and intestinal contents have provided insight into the way these people lived. From our point of view, what is interesting was that one of the women had lungs full of soot and another had a large nasal cancer that had spread to surrounding areas, possibly rendering her blind in one eye and deaf. More organic combustibles damaging the airways in a uniquely human way; airways that did not evolve with this kind of assault in mind. More delayed penalties to set against the benefits of pyromania?

There are yet more striking examples of cancers attributable to products of carboniferous combustion that I want to relate, but these are more appropriately considered in another context. Now it's time to cool off.

CHAPTER 15

WOMEN'S TROUBLES

You can seldom find a convent that does not harbour this accursed pest, cancer, within its walls.

(Bernardino Ramazzini, 1700, with reference to breast cancer)

Sex was invented not, as the poet Philip Larkin mused, in 1963, but a very long time ago. The first conjugal union between two different members of a unicellular species was a chance coupling some 3000 million years ago. They fused, shared, and shifted their genes and the world became a different place. When I sat the undergraduate entrance exams for the Zoology Department at University College London in the early 1960s, a question posed by John Maynard Smith, one of the UK's leading evolutionary biologists, was: 'Is sex necessary?' It had never occurred to me that this could be an issue. The answer goes along the lines that sexual reproduction is really about mixing and shuffling of parental genes. This serves to both create extra genetic diversity in offspring and ensure that not all offspring inherit any deleterious mutations lurking in the germ line. The pay-off of this genetic versatility is better survival prospects (for at least some offspring). Survival in a forever changing, hostile, and parasite-ridden world is the gist of what many biologists believe the invention of sex was really all about, although the argument is richer and more complex than this.

Whatever the evolutionary logic, we can be confident that sex in the good old days equated with reproduction. Flowering plants do it, worms do it in hermaphroditic couplings, large marine mammals miraculously manage it. Now I'm not going to contend that we are the only species that is motivated by pleasure in this context, since it almost certainly isn't true. What does seem to be exceptional for higher primates, and especially *Homo sapiens*, is the progressive divorce between sex and reproduction and our social manipulation of these two activities. Other than our close relative, the bonobo or pygmy chimpanzee, we are unique in the exploitation of sex as recreation rather than procreation. Natural as this may seem, sex and reproduction are deeply embedded together in our genetic heritage. But we have decoupled these activities in a manner that no other species has or can do, and have done so by

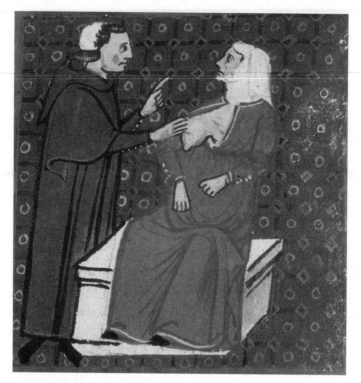

Figure 15.1 Examination of the breast by the surgeon, Teodorico Borgognoni (1275). See also colour plate section.

rapid social means that largely escape the Darwinian filter or test of genetic fitness. Cancer may be one major if indirect consequence of this.

La femme est une malade

Women get a particularly bad deal in the cancer stakes and have done so for a long time. This is reflected in both historical accounts and current incidence rates that portray a high frequency of cancers in the female reproductive system (the ovary, uterus, cervix) and particularly in the breast. A raw deal not only in the risk of cancer but also in the treatment itself. The loss of a breast, such an entrenched symbol of womanhood, is bad enough but the sheer crudity and indignity of the would-be remedies in historical times was simply awful. Blood-sucking leeches and frogs compete in the medieval lexicon along with potions in which, inexplicably, excrement of rats, goats, or men, feature prominently. And then there was surgery.

It's difficult, if not impossible, for us to imagine what it must have been like before the days of anaesthetics, hygienic and reparative surgery, and antibiotics to suffer an amputation and cauterization. Historical surgical tests provide graphic illustrations of instrumentation and methods and a macabre hint at what was involved. The closest we can get to the reality of surgery for breast cancer in earlier times is to read a record of it by a woman who was both an accomplished writer and a patient – Fanny Burney. Her graphic account, written to her sister in 1811, is a tribute to her remarkable stoicism and a chilling catalogue of indignity and pain incurred. Against the odds, Fanny Burney lived for another 30 years after her surgery. Mastectomy has remained the mainstay of breast cancer treatment for two thousand years and the fact that surgical methods have greatly improved scarcely disguises what is at best a crude and partially effective remedy; a testament to our failures. Only now it's on offer as a prophylactic measure too. Radical bilateral mastectomy in healthy women with a family history of breast cancer has been reported to prevent 90 per cent of predicted cases. Somehow this leaves me unimpressed. The price for silence is high and anyway not every woman in such families is at risk.

Breast cancer has been a predominant type of cancer for centuries, at least in Europe, and steadily increased in incidence throughout the twentieth century in Westernized countries, long before man-made DDT or radiation, petrochemical industries, and corporation culture came to dominate the scene. Currently, the risk or probability of an American or European female having a diagnosis of breast cancer is close to 1 in 10. Note however that this alarming statistic is somewhat inflated by detection by screening for clinically silent cancers that may never have emerged and that the figure is not only an average but reflects the cumulative lifetime risk for those living to be 85 years old. Cardiovascular disease poses a greater threat. Also, although a significant minority of patients with breast cancer will be relatively young or pre-menopausal, most are older. The risk of a 30-year-old woman developing breast cancer during the following decade is down at a 1 in 250 chance. Surgical treatment, adjutant chemotherapy, screening and early diagnosis, and overall patient management have also improved greatly and a substantial proportion of patients benefit from long-term remission or cure. But, something is obviously very wrong here. An awful number of relatively young to middle-aged women do develop breast cancer and even more have silent and incipient cancers that never see the light of day. Why have mammary glands become a minefield of genetic mishaps?

Artefacts recovered from the remains of Greek temples suggest that in the years before Hippocrates, Greeks would place clay models of breast tumours as votives in temples in the vain hope that an illness of supposed supernatural cause might be remedied by supernatural intervention (Fig. 15.2). Hippocrates and his Cos school of surgeon-physicians, and later Galen, regarded breast cancer as a by-product of a melancholic predisposition. This quasi-scientific or

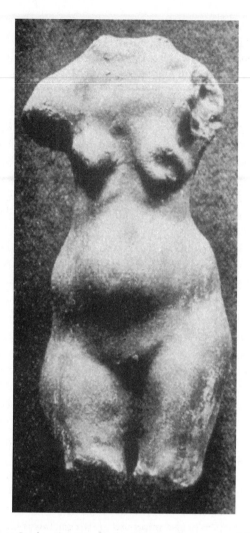

Figure 15.2 Ancient Greek votive statuette showing ulcerating tumour of the breast.

rather pseudo-scientific view proved extraordinarily tenacious and greatly exercised the minds of more recent medicine men. Take for example Herbert Snow, distinguished surgeon at the Cancer Hospital in London where I now work and who used, but didn't coin, the pithy French aphorism that serves as our subtitle. Writing his essays towards the end of the nineteenth century, Snow personifies the Victorian gentleman's talent for appearing polite, pompous, and patronizing at the same time. Snow noted that cancer was a characteristic feature of 'civilised communities' that lacked what he believed to be 'the immunity of savage races, lunatics and idiots'. In an essay beginning

'Gentlemen ...', Snow announced that the proclivity of women to develop cancer, particularly of the breast and uterus, was due to the debilitated lifestyle and neuroses of civilized women. This was reflected in their 'proneness to constipation, abuse of neurotics (sic) such as tea' but most significantly in terms of tumour causation to 'the universal habit amongst civilised women in Europe and the USA of wearing bodily constricting corsets from a young age'. On the same theme of undergarments and cancer, the gloriously named Clot Bey suggested that the rarity of uterine cancer amongst Egyptian women was due to the wearing of drawers which protected the genital region from eddies of cold air.

Snow, along with other eminent eighteenth- and nineteenth-century cancer surgeons in England, France, and the USA, actively promulgated the view, originating many centuries before, that the root cause lay in women's psyche exacerbated perhaps by chronic irritation (physical irritation, that is). The sub-plot that breast cancer arises as a consequence of grief was also firmly entrenched in the surgical spirit of the day. The evidence was, to say the least, anecdotal. Here are quotes on two of the cases preferred as supporting the thesis:

> Case 1: The Wife of a Mate of a Ship (who was taken some Time ago by the French, and put in Prison) was thereby so much affected, that her breast began to swell, and soon after broke out in a desperate cancer which had proceeded so far that I could not undertake her case. She never before had any complaint in her breast.
>
> *(Richard Guy, 1759)*
>
> Case 2: Emma B., aged 49; single. No family history; no blow or injury. School mistress. Has had more or less trouble for years; had a carbuncle on the shoulder three years ago; and has not felt strong since. Has been much over-worked at school. Says that last June she felt almost out of her mind, and was ready to throw herself out of the window. Father was ill in bed for six months last year; had much anxiety about him, and for several months at the beginning of 1883 pecuniary troubles. The tumours appeared about Christmas last.
>
> (Herbert Snow, 1883)

It is alarming to consider that prominent surgeons could indulge in such nonsense. But the idea still retains a curious holistic appeal to some, despite lack of any credible evidence or plausible biological mechanism. Systematic studies in the 1960s, 70s, and 80s found no consistent and significant associations between breast cancer and prior stressful events and there is no evidence persuasively linking breast cancer causation with attributes of personality. Even if there were to be, as suggested by a few studies, some averaged differences in long-standing behavioural features of breast cancer patients versus controls, this need not imply causality. Psychosomatic depression of the immune system is very unlikely to be a contributory factor. Women whose immunological defences have been profoundly compromised by medical treatment, as transplant recipients for example, are not at extra risk of breast cancer.

Other eighteenth- and nineteenth-century surgeons, including distinguished British surgeons John Hunter and James Paget, believed that breast and other cancers could follow soon after a physical blow or trauma in individuals who were constitutionally predisposed. The constitutional argument appears to be based both on clinical impressions of cancer-prone families and, in particular, on the observation that following surgery for the primary cancer, the disease would usually or relentlessly reappear in some other part of the body. Clearly there was no appreciation of the inherent latency of cancer and, rather more surprisingly, an apparent ignorance of metastatic spread. The French, it has to be said, were better informed!

The often quoted remark by Bernardino Ramazzini at the start of this chapter may move us somewhat nearer to reality and it's worth looking at his comments in full:

> But where there is no placenta to be considered, as in the case of virgins who sometimes generate milk in the breasts, we must still admit this sympathy between the breasts and uterus; for experience proves that as a consequence of disturbances in the uterus, cancerous tumors are very often generated in women's breasts, and tumors of this sort are found in nuns more than in any other women. Now these are not caused by suppression of the menses but rather, in my opinion, by their celibate life. For I have known several cases of nuns who came to a pitiable end from terrible cancers of the breasts; these women had healthy complexions, and their menses occurred regularly, but they were born wantons. Every city in Italy has several religious communities of nuns, and you can seldom find a convent that does not harbor this accursed pest, cancer, within its walls. Now why is it that the breasts suffer for the derangements of the womb, whereas other parts of the body do not suffer in this way or not so frequently? It is certainly because there is between them a mysterious sympathy that so far has escaped the researches of prosectors, though perhaps the course of time will reveal it, since the whole domain of Truth has not yet been conquered.

Losing to an own goal?

There isn't a universal or single cause for breast cancer. And frustratingly, in individual cases, causation is likely to remain elusive or at least beyond the grasp of certainty. The only known causal mechanism is ionizing radiation, but this only accounts for a small minority of cases. However, the best bet for explaining most breast as well as uterine (endometrial) and ovarian cancers may be that they reflect a major 'own goal' or hormonal penalty for being human and female. An own goal inadvertently but effectively energized by changes in diet and lifestyle. Best bet in this author's personal view plus that of some, but by no means all, epidemiologists who have studied the problem directly. I won't give you all the caveats that are endemic to epidemiological investigations of disease. The proferred explanation makes much sense when seen in an evolutionary context and may lead eventually to effective preventive measures. Maybe, if correct, the mechanism will only account for some, but not all, cases and maybe it is prudent to call it a theory with the appendage of a question mark, but the magnitude and urgency of the problem requires that some shrewd bets be taken now.

The stark reality is that females of our species are burdened with a five-million-year-old genetic programme that anatomically and physiologically primes them for regular pregnancy and lactation. But then our rapid social development as a species has produced a schism between our socialized re-productive behaviour and our evolutionary heritage – nature and nurture in conflict. Epidemiologists argue over the strength of the risk factors associated with breast cancer but the long-standing observations by Ramazzini and others in Italy and France that this cancer was common in convent nuns provided an early clue. In his ground-breaking survey of mortality from cancer in Verona from 1760 to 1839, Rigoni-Stern found that nuns were five times more likely to die of cancer than married women and that the former had a considerable excess of breast cancer plus a deficit of uterine (cervical?) cancer. His original paper also reveals another rather extraordinary and neglected fact. His four cases of male breast cancer were all in priests as was the first case recorded of male breast cancer by British physician John of Arderne in the fourteenth century. Rigoni-Stern proferred no explanation for this bizarre observation[3] but neither had he a clue about the reason for the connection with religious sisters. Reflecting contemporary ideas on mechanical stress and cancer, he did ask if the high rate of breast cancer might not be attributable to the wearing of tight habits or 'perhaps, the long sustained bent position assumed while saying prayers with forearms resting on knees and compressing the breasts'. Rigoni-Stern also knew that unmarried spinsters were more at risk of breast cancer, so it perhaps is surprising that he didn't reflect on what they and nuns had in common. I suspect he would also miss the boat if he was around today and knew that breast cancer has a low incidence in Aborigine populations, multiparous women generally, female athletes, and ballet dancers.

Our female ovulatory cycle, along with that of our closest primate relatives – the gorilla, chimpanzee, and orang-utan, is programmed for 35 years or so of constant, non-seasonal activity. Breaks before menopause are applied only in pregnancy and during lactation. The ovarian hormones – oestradiol (the major oestrogen) and progesterone – are secreted into the blood during timed phases of the ovulatory cycle and impinge on breast tissue. The ductal epithelium of breasts is then under a monthly pulse of hormonal inducement to proliferate – primed in anticipation of pregnancy and demand for suckling. The epithelium of the ovary and uterine endometrium are similarly subject to monthly wound repair and regenerative stress following each cycle of ovulation.

Since most other primates in the wild have the more conventional arrangement of seasonal fluctuation in oestra, we can assume that programming constant ovulation and mammary gland priming is a relatively recent evolutionary adaptation, say 15 million years or so (somewhere near the base of the great ape tree of which we are a side branch). One can conjure up plausible though untestable explanations as to why this might have had selective advantage. For example, most mammals time seasonal ovulation via light cues in order to ensure that offspring have sufficient food, water, and warmth. Rhesus monkeys have a seasonal ovulatory cycle in the wild but constantly cycle when in zoos where seasonal variation in light, temperature, and food supplies are, to a large extent, neutralized. One might imagine that as our Hominid predecessors emerged out of Africa and ventured beyond the tropics, they will have encountered climatic conditions that might have favoured seasonal restriction of reproduction (the rhesus monkey move in reverse). But then there would have been a counter pressure. Once humans, or hominid predecessors, developed effective strategies for provision of food, water, warmth (fire again!), and shelter, there would be a potential reproductive advantage for any females that could conceive at any time of year. The great ape pattern of ovulatory cycles would therefore be retained or reinstated. Genetic changes that directly enhance reproductive success generally earn high adaptive currency in the evolutionary stakes.

Comparisons of the reproductive biology of modern women, say in the USA or Scandinavia, with those in contemporary hunter-gatherer or Aborigine societies, allow some estimates to be made of the impact of lifestyle on the oestrogen pump and potential cancer risk. Figure 15.3 is a visual presentation to aid the discussion that follows. It illustrates the stark differences in reproductive habits and concomitant ovarian oestrogen pump activity that are the inevitable correlates of our social advances. Primitive Eve may have been programmed for regular menstrual cycles, and fertile, between say age 17 and 45. Regular pregnancy and an average of six births plus lactation (lasting say a total of three years each) might be expected to inhibit more than 200 cycles. Four hundred potential cycles might be reduced to around 150 on average and, along with it, proliferative stress and risk to ovarian tissue and the breast. But there's the rub. Since antiquity, women have resisted this biological set-up.

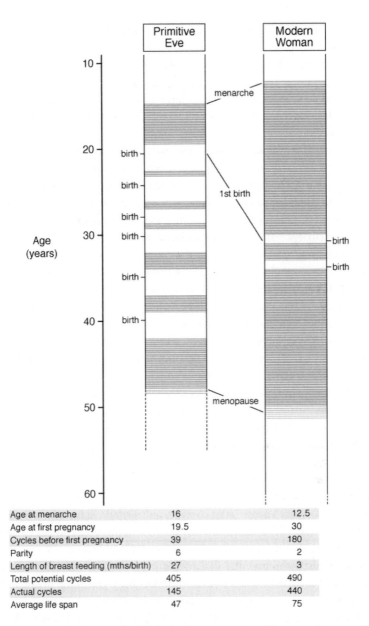

	Primitive Eve	Modern Woman
Age at menarche	16	12.5
Age at first pregnancy	19.5	30
Cycles before first pregnancy	39	180
Parity	6	2
Length of breast feeding (mths/birth)	27	3
Total potential cycles	405	490
Actual cycles	145	440
Average life span	47	75

Figure 15.3 An evolutionary cycle ride. A visual representation of the approximate number of monthly ovulatory cycles (and pulses of oestrogen/progesterone to the breast epithelium) in early versus modern (Westernised) woman. 'Primitive Eve' data based upon recent observations of women in hunter-gatherer tribes (1 in 6 births assumed to have resulted in neonatal death). Each horizontal line represents one cycle. Dotted lines represent irregular cycles and lower oestrogen levels.

Historically, the process of change has been slow and accumulative. First, fewer pregnancies. As women began to exercise the option of choice and males of the species showed a modicum of restraint or selectivity, there will have been cohorts of women with fewer or no pregnancies. Hence the increased risk of breast and ovarian cancer linked to a life of religious celibacy, affluence, or higher social class and the sustained low risk of multiparous but poor women in the developing countries. In more modern societies, the relevant trends would have been towards later pregnancy. Less directly, dietary changes including greater calorie consumption plus a more sedentary lifestyle (that is, less burning of calories) have led to a progressive lowering of the age of puberty and sustained higher oestrogen levels, as I will return to shortly. These changes are believed to conspire together to increase the number of ovulatory cycles women experience and the proliferative stress to the breast, as well as to the uterine endometrium and ovary itself.

A large fraction of women in the USA and Europe now delay their first child until their late twenties or early thirties and an increasing number have no children at all. This, combined with an earlier start to puberty and ovarian and menstrual cycles (menarche) – averaging 12.5 years in the USA compared with 16 years in hunter-gatherer societies – guarantees that for a woman having her first child at age 30 years, around 200 oestrogenic cycles have occurred since puberty. In less developed societies, and we assume for early humans as for pongo, pan, and other higher primate relatives, the gap or number of menstrual cycles between post-pubertal fertility and first pregnancy is relatively brief (around 2.5 years or 30 cycles of ovulation (see Fig. 15.3). This is the biological norm with respect to our genetic programming that reflects prior evolutionary adaptations to very different social conditions.

The hormonal trap has been worsened still more by changes in breast-feeding habits. Breast-feeding for two to three years was the norm for most women in ancient Egypt, India, Greece, and Rome, endorsed by Talmudic texts, the Koran, and social traditions. Early hominids probably continued the practice of prolonged nurture and breast-feeding on demand that is a feature of other higher primates. In rural African communities today, where breast cancer is rare, 18 months or more of breast-feeding is common. Breast-feeding practices have probably varied considerably throughout human development in relation to availability of alternative foods, social structures, and other factors, but in so far as it is possible to define a 'natural' timing for weaning, it is probably between two and four years.

The benefits to the infant of breast-feeding and breast milk have long been recognized and for this reason, when wealthier women declined to breast-feed (in ancient Greece or later in eighteenth-century Europe) wet nurses were co-opted to provide the service. The benefit for the suckling infant comes in the form of bonding and, via milk itself, nutritional and immunological support during a fragile period. What does it do for mum? Suckling at the nipple induces prolactin hormone production which in turn restrains further ovulation. The adaptive advantage of this arrangement could be that it allowed primitive Eve to provide full succour to her immature infants without the diversion of another pregnancy, and to avoid what might otherwise be continuous pregnancy. That this reflects an early adaptation of *Homo sapiens* cannot be proved but is indirectly supported by observations on the !Kung tribe. These hunter-gatherers of Namibia and Botswana are regarded by some anthropologists as having a lifestyle and social organization resembling that of our Stone Age predecessors in the Pleistocene period. The average birth spacing in this group is 44 months, which at one time was regarded as a puzzle since the group did not indulge in celibacy and was not familiar with contraception. Nutritional insufficiency might have been the explanation but it probably isn't. It turns out that this interval of infertility is correlated with prolonged breast-feeding and a reduction in blood serum levels of those hormones that stimulate gonadal function and ovulation (oestradiol and progesterone).

The same story applies to other Aborigine populations. The Gainj people are tribal highlanders in Papua New Guinea. A study of their reproductive habits revealed a similar pattern of prolonged breast-feeding and a likely impact on reducing ovulatory cycles and increasing birth spacing. In this reproductive respect, the Aborigine groups behave similarly to wild orang-utans, gorillas, and chimpanzees, and we assume have a reproductive lifestyle relatively unchanged from the earliest *Homo sapiens* – and one that is commensurate with prior adaptation and selection in the great apes. We've become rather different in style in the intervening five million years, but not in genetics.

Changes in breast-feeding habits were particularly dramatic in the twentieth century. Concomitant with social advances, changes in employment practices, and contraceptive use, women *en masse* reduced breast-feeding to a minimum. In the USA and Europe, most mothers breast-feed either briefly or for three to six months according to circumstances and to some extent fashion. Under these circumstances, there will be a rapid return to ovarian activity, fertility, and monthly hormonal stress to the breast.

Breast-feeding will certainly reduce the physiological stress that operates via ovarian secretion of oestradiol and progesterone hormones, but there may well be more local mechanisms of protection at work as well. Chinese Tanka or boat people in southern China and Hong Kong traditionally breast-feed their infants unilaterally (with the right breast only). In these women, the risk of breast cancer post-menopausally has been reported to be significantly more likely to occur, if it occurs at all, in the unsuckled breast. There is a similar suggestion that amongst Canadian Inuit women, the unsuckled breast is most at risk of cancer. Observations such as these need to be repeated to be credible but they provide yet another indication or reminder that we have much still to learn about our physiology.

But then the explanation of why an early pregnancy, independently of number of pregnancies, should be protective against breast cancer is not entirely clear. We know from studies on women who developed breast cancer as a consequence of exposure to ionizing radiation either 'accidentally' (the atomic bomb in Japan) or therapeutically (for scalp ringworm or of the chest region for Hodgkin's disease, for example) that very young females aged 5 to 15 were most at risk. Although breast cancer is not normally initiated by ionizing radiation, this observation is probably telling us that the critical stem cells in the breast are most active in this peripubertal period (for which there is some experimental evidence). One possible explanation for the protective effect of an early pregnancy is then that it resets the timetable or programme of activity for these crucial cells – for example by forcing cell differentiation out of the stem cell compartment – thereby reducing the number of cells 'at risk'.

Risk of radiation therapy-induced breast cancer declines with age at exposure, concomitant with changes in breast physiology. Seen in this light, it is not surprising that the very marked socially driven changes in the interval between first full ovulatory cycle and first pregnancy (see Fig. 15.3) have a significant impact on cancer risk. Paradoxically, women with a late first pregnancy seem to be more at risk than those with no pregnancy at all. Pregnancy itself provides a massive stimulation for ductal epithelium proliferation in the breast (as a prelude to lactation) and one possibility is that this stimulus, if occurring later in life, may promote the development of cancerous cells that have already arisen earlier following persistent stimulation of very many cycles of proliferative stress.

Now go back and look at Fig. 15.3. The overall impact of social changes in reproductive habits that slowly accrued over the past 5000 years and accelerated in the twentieth century in developed societies, have been dramatic in two important biological respects: first, the continuation of cycles of hormonal secretion for years without a break following puberty and, second, the total accumulation of cycles and hormone exposure between the ages of 15 and 50 years. With some imagination and taking some liberties, we could redraw Fig. 15.3 on a sliding scale and so place, in between the two extremes shown, the 'average' woman of ancient Greece, eighteenth-century European woman, current Japanese woman (living in Japan), nulliparous nuns, or women of different social classes in western society at different times. It has been a sliding scale and slippery slope of risk for quite some time but the last hundred years has witnessed an acceleration.

Regrettably there's still more to be concerned about. The internal oestrogen pump is being supplemented from outside. Some of the high-dose oestrogen pills that were taken by many women starting in the early 1960s have, for those who took them for prolonged periods, increased risk still further. Unfortunately we may now be in the process of making matters even worse as far as breast cancer is concerned. We shouldn't be too surprised to see recent research suggesting that oestrogen-based HRT for post-menopausal women may significantly increase, albeit modestly, the risk of breast cancer – though, when combined with progesterone, it may actually decrease the risk of endometrial cancer of the uterus. At the same time, the epidemiological data are somewhat contentious and there are other clear benefits to be derived from HRT. This raises the spectre of some difficult choices facing women: do you want to run what may be up to a 50 per cent increased risk of having breast cancer but feel good, look good, be more mentally alert, and have a reduced chance of dying of endometrial cancer, heart disease, or suffering from osteoporosis?

Environmental chemicals with oestrogenic activity have also been attracting suspicion, especially in the USA. There are a plethora of substances with weak oestrogenic or antioestrogenic activity but those considered to have criminal credentials include the organochlorine pesticide DDT and the industrial polychlorinated biphenyls (PCBs). Concerns here are exacerbated by tales of the feminization of male animals and falling sperm counts in men. These chemicals, when consumed, can be concentrated and then persist in fat tissue. They can have oestrogen-like activity in stimulating breast cancer cells in a test-tube, but whether the concentrations of such molecules ever approaches that required to have a real impact on breast cancer risk is, however, far from clear. Moreover, epidemiological studies have so far failed to demonstrate any convincing or consistent association with breast cancer. So the jury is still out on this one. The psychology of this situation is however interesting – the desire to regard a weak xeno-oestrogen, with its industrial parentage, as a villain whilst one's own endogenous hormones by their 'natural' status must be accredited innocence. A form of xenophobia maybe, when the problem is really closer to home?

The indirect epidemiological evidence supporting the hormonal stress theory, particularly in relation to reproductive habits, is persuasive though inevitably incomplete. The first epidemiological evidence implicating reproductive events (or the lack of them) derived from a case versus controls study in the UK provided by Janet Lane-Claypon in 1926. A great deal of data have been assembled since that time but more direct or experimental evidence is difficult to come by. It's been known for over a hundred years that removal of the oestrogen source (ovaries) drastically reduces the risk of breast cancer but this would still be compatible with other exogenous factors mutating hormone-dependent cells in the proliferating breast. It's not a lot better than saying that breast cancer in men is very rare. More than 60 years ago, researchers showed that continual administration of oestrogen to mice induced mammary cancer. This has a tragic but revealing human parallel. Two cases of breast cancer have been recorded in transsexual men who had been treated for five years with large doses of oestrogen.

In most cases of breast cancer, the sustained proliferative activity of the malignant cells is dependent upon oestrogens, which is why ovary ablation was originally employed as a therapeutic tactic and modern regimens use anti-oestrogen drugs. With progression and metastasis of disease, the cancer clone often becomes independent of its oestrogenic stimulus. This is usually because antioestrogen therapy has supplied the selective pressure for a mutant oestrogen-independent subclone to emerge (the classical Darwinian mechanism of drug resistance). Other observations on animals are revealing and I'm impressed by what happens with domestic poultry. These birds have been selected for constant egg production and it is unlikely to be coincidental that ovarian adenocarcinoma is their commonest epithelial cancer. More strikingly, if their egg production rate is stepped up by twelve hours' artificial light a day, then the majority, as reported in one study, develop ovarian cancer. If hens really had breasts, the story would be even more persuasive.

Turning the ratchet

So is that all it is – too much oestrogen and progesterone from constantly cycling ovaries? Why is it Japanese women had enjoyed a relatively low rate of breast cancer but rates have doubled in Japan since 1945 and approach high Western rates one generation after emigration to the USA? Why is height a risk factor for breast cancer? Adoption of Western diets is one very plausible explanation, especially as dietary habits when young impact on menstrual cycles and hormone levels. Most Japanese women back home still have menarche at a later age, have lower average oestrogen levels, and partake of relatively low-fat diets with modest total calorie intakes compared with their USA counterparts. Dietary studies on breast cancer have not produced consistent results, particularly with respect to fat intake, but the overall trend in Westernized cultures from Hawaii to Norway is for excess calories to be linked to extra risk, perhaps along with a deficiency of antioxidant-rich foods. Some regular ingredients of oriental cuisine (soy in particular) may also lower oestrogen levels and consumption of these has been associated in some epidemiological studies with a lowered risk of breast cancer. Extra calorie intake by girls may be linked to earlier menarche (as observed in offspring of Japanese immigrants to the USA) and to higher oestrogen levels in adults.

The interplay of dietary intake and exercise, or relative lack of it, and the resultant energy balance is also likely to be important. In this respect, it is interesting that female athletes and ballet dancers have a relatively high rate of amenorrhoea (lack of regular periods), a later menarche, and a reported lower risk of breast cancer. Excess, unburnt calories can also provide the energy drive for more cell proliferation and more oxidative stress to cells, in the breast and elsewhere. One important player in this physiological game has been attracting attention recently. Excess calorie intake and increased size and/or weight are associated with increased levels in the circulation of a hormone called insulin-like growth factor 1 or IGF-1. This is one of our key general regulators of cell behaviour and not only promotes cell proliferation but inhibits cell death – in other words, a powerful promoter of clonal expansion. Some scientists believe it could be a key modulator of cancer risk, not only for breast cancer but for prostate and other common subtypes that appear to be influenced by diet and lifestyle.

So, do me a favour and look back once again at Fig. 15.3. If we equate the continuity and total number of monthly ovarian hormone signals to the breast as pulses of risk, then I should draw the lines two or three times the thickness for our 'Modern Woman' to reflect the likely impact of raised blood levels of oestradiol and IGF-1.

More fat may be bad news on other scores. In post-menopausal women, the ovarian oestrogen tap is turned off but fat tissue contains enzymes that can generate oestrogens from other tissue sources. A high fat intake has also been linked in experimental studies to promotion of a metabolic pathway that converts oestradiol to a product, hydroxyoestrone, that may be directly genotoxic or DNA-damaging. Some recent research indicates that breast fat can act as a sponge or absorbent for mutagenic substances, which has set alarm bells ringing.

On the whole, however, there is very little convincing or consistent evidence that breast cancer is associated with exposure to recognized external carcinogens. There is a hint that, for some women, smoking may increase the risk of breast cancer but the effect is marginal and other reports even suggest that smoking might confer some degree of protection via antioestrogenic effects. Despite the rabid toxicity of tobacco's combustion products, they do not appear to exert much of an impact on breast cancer rates. Risk of breast cancer does increase, though over a modest twofold range, with alcohol intake. It's unclear how alcohol achieves this effect but it's more likely to be via hormonal changes than direct carcinogenicity.

Conceiving a risk

The risk of breast and ovarian cancer is subject to yet one other variable – the genetic lottery that is held at the moment of conception. Human populations carry at least two genes that strongly predispose towards breast or breast plus ovarian cancer when inherited in a mutant form. These are referred to as *BRCA-1* and *BRCA-2*. Following their identification by molecular cloning, these genes attracted widespread publicity, partly because of the very competitive arena in which their discovery was made, priority disputes, and the potential for commercial exploitation but also, quite appropriately, because of their marked biological impact and predictive implications.

Around 5 to 10 per cent of all breast or ovarian cancers show familial clustering and are likely to involve inherited genes. Somewhat less than half of these involve *BRCA-1* or *BRCA-2*, so other renegade genes await detection. But for those women that have a mutant variety of the *BRCA-1* or *BRCA-2* gene, around 60 per cent will develop breast cancer and 15 per cent, ovarian cancer. And, paradoxically, pregnancies actually *increase* the risk of breast cancer for women who are carriers of *BRCA-1* or *BRCA-2* genes. These patients will also tend to develop their cancers at an earlier age than other patients. One implication of this is that quite a sizeable fraction of breast cancers below the age of 35 years may involve constitutive or inherited mutant genes. And as some will be new mutants in the germ line, not all young cases will have a prior family history of breast cancer. In this context, it's clearly of some importance to try and identify other genes that may be kick-starting breast cancer in young women.

The risk for breast cancer is therefore high in females who by an accident of history inherit a mutant *BRCA* gene from either their mother or father; high enough to persuade some to opt for a radical double mastectomy – high, but not inevitable. There are now pairs of identical twins carrying the same *BRCA* gene mutation in whom one has had breast cancer but the other, many years later, has not, despite experiencing a similar reproductive history. Chance rears its head again – this time in the probability of one or more of the essential additional and non-inherited mutations occurring. A few male offspring may also develop breast cancer, as well as having a higher risk of prostate cancer, if they inherit a mutant *BRCA-2* gene.

We all inherit normal or innocent *BRCA-1* and *BRCA-2* genes but on average about 1 in 800 of us carry one of these two genes in a mutant form, and this figure is higher still for some groups – 1 in 50 for Ashkenazi Jews for example. Such a high frequency of a dangerous gene requires an explanation. It is certainly much greater than can be explained by mutation rate considerations. It is also difficult to imagine how, historically, those carrying the mutation could have had a reproductive advantage, as in the case of mutations in the β-haemoglobin gene in black Africans that is associated with sickle cell anaemia but confers the benefit of protection from malaria. One would expect the opposite if anything, with gene carriers being at a selective disadvantage.

Over 140 different mutant forms of the *BRCA-1* and *BRCA-2* genes have already been identified. These will have arisen independently but one mutant form only will be shared within a family. In contrast, only two or three unique and common mutations are found in Ashkenazi Jews. In Iceland, families with excess cases of breast and ovarian cancers have the same single and unique *BRCA-2* gene mutation. In contrast, Italian families have a range of different mutations. The most likely explanation for the predominance and prevalence of particular mutant genes in populations is via what evolutionary biologist, Ernst Mayer, termed the 'founder effect'. This is a situation shared by species of microbes, plants, animals, and man where a large group of individuals has been derived historically from a very small number of predecessors and remains relatively isolated, such that any unusual gene in the starting pool can be represented at an appreciable frequency in the descendants. In a few instances, a common mutant and associated disease in a geographically restricted community can be backtracked to a single, named individual – as in the case of Miss Cundick, an English immigrant to Tasmania, who innocently imported a mutant gene for Huntington's disease in 1848.

This then suggests that the derivation of at least some current Ashkenazi populations was from a small number of individuals, probably in central or eastern Europe, one of whom happened by accident to acquire an inheritable *BRCA-1* mutation in his or her germ cells.

Gene mutations with a relatively high prevalence are likely to have originated very many generations ago. The most common *BRCA-1* mutation in Russia and Europe generally is thought to have originated in the Baltic region some 38 generations ago, in the eleventh century. One of the two most common *BRCA-1* mutations in Ashkenazi Jews is shared with Jewish families in Iran and Iraq. Since these populations separated some 2000 years ago, it has been suggested that the nameless founding individual in whom the mutation first arose lived before that period. It may seem odd that a gene carrying a variable but generally high risk of a lethal illness can persist down through so many generations. But it can do so if carriers have offspring before they become seriously ill or die of other causes or if they remain healthy, as will some mothers and even more fathers. And this essentially is what has happened, and continues to occur both with ancient and new mutations in *BRCA* genes.

Clearly *BRCA-1* and *BRCA-2* genes encode functions that impact in a powerful way on the stem cells of the breast, ovarian, and other epithelia. How they do so is currently a topic of intense research. The terminology for these genes is perhaps misleading in this context. Inheritance of a mutant *BRCA-2* gene increases the risk of not only breast and ovarian cancers but cancers of the prostate, stomach, and pancreas. Some critical but broad cell regulating function must be involved. The proteins encoded by these genes look as though they may be involved both in DNA repair and cell proliferation. By the time this book is published, we will probably know exactly what they do.

Other genes predisposing to breast cancer certainly exist, including *p53* in families with the Li-Fraumeni syndrome and *PTEN* in Cowden syndrome. Overall, the chance inheritance of a *mutant* gene probably accounts for some 5 to 10 per cent of all breast cancers but this still represents a large number of patients. Issues of genetic screening for these mutations, risk prediction, counselling, and prophylactic intervention are therefore understandably important and contentious topics of much current debate.

Other genes inherited in a normal but variable form (and function) may act indirectly to modify risk of breast cancer. The relatively high concordance rate of breast cancer in twins (around 25% for those that are monozygotic or identical) provides a hint that inherited genetics other than mutant genes may be important. It would be very surprising if the genetic circuits regulating oestrogen hormone signalling were not subject to intrinsic or inherited variation. Recent research indeed suggests that women inheriting normal variants of genes that influence oestrogen metabolism are at increased risk of breast cancer. Any genetic variants promoting fertility would have been at an evolutionary advantage in earlier times. Increased risk of breast cancer could be the ironic flip side of this adaptive coin. The potentially deleterious trade-off would, however, lie dormant and untranslated into real risk until such times as behavioural modulation of hormonal circuits teased out the underlying design flaw.

A synopsis of 'cause'

I want to finish this section with two general but important biological considerations of breast cancer: the time frame over which the cancer clone develops and a distillation of what the 'cause' may be.

Risk generally increases with age over several decades between 20 and 70 years, but the rate of increase slows down after menopause. The average age of a woman with breast cancer will be just a few years after menopause. It may have been similarly so in ancient Greece as Hippocrates noted an association of the onset of cancer with the cessation of menstruation. But the average age at diagnosis is derived from a broad range and is not very helpful when it comes to understanding the time frame of the critical biological events. From our current view of the clonal evolution of cancer, we would anticipate a protracted period of cancer formation. Studies on cohorts of women who developed breast cancer as a consequence of radiation exposure suggest that the gap or latency between an initial DNA-damaging event and subsequent malignancy averages around 20 years, with an increased risk persisting for 50 years in individuals exposed when very young.

Malignant breast cancer will be preceded by the presence of so-called atypical ductal hyperplasia or one or more small tumours which are, in themselves, benign. These may (or may not) progress to localized 'carcinomas *in situ*' (CIS) which in turn may evolve into invasive breast cancer (or more often do not). Prospective or serial monitoring studies on large numbers of women having breast biopsies have suggested 10 to 15-year intervals for breast cancer to emerge through this key bottleneck in clonal evolution. So, for a woman of 50 with breast cancer, we can at least hazard a guess at when the first mutation happened or when the eventually dominant clone first began to emerge as a mutant. It seems likely that this key event occurs relatively early in life, although we have no way yet of pinning it down. Indeed of the various acquired (non-inherited) genetic abnormalities detected in breast cancer cells, we don't know which one comes first. It is certainly possible that the early mutational events occur predominantly in the years immediately following puberty but we know from the awful experience of the Japanese atomic bomb that the process can start at as young as five years. Breast stem cells are in fact generated during foetal development in the womb and the suggestion has been made that the first DNA mishaps could even occur then, to be revealed only much later when oestrogen drive kicks in.

We don't know but the answer is likely to be that the evolutionary trail of clonal escape in breast cancer starts early in life and normally takes decades to emerge. The conclusion to draw is that the risk level for breast cancer later in life is almost certainly modulated during the teenage years; set up, but not necessarily hard-wired.

So what, in this context, is the 'cause' of breast cancer? There really is no argument that endogenous hormonal effects on the breast, dictated in some considerable measure by reproductive history, diet, and exercise, are playing a key role. Critics of this view argue that the increased risk levels derived from epidemiological studies are relatively modest and therefore these factors can together only account, collectively, for a maximum of somewhere between 50 and 60 per cent of risk. Unfortunately, we expect more of epidemiology than it can provide in this context. There is no simple way of computing the cumulative impact of oestradiol, progesterone, and IGF-1 levels in breast epithelium cell turnover in individual women over several decades. It's naïve to expect retrospectively assessed indices of lifestyle, particularly when diet and exercise are concerned, to provide accurate risk estimates. We therefore do not know, and cannot know for sure, what the actual risk of breast cancer is from general measures of reproductive and menstrual history, diet, and exercise.[4] Everything suggests that it is substantial and even if it were to be only 50 per cent, which I doubt, then that would be worth writing home about. Wouldn't it?

Some scientists hold the view that whilst chronic hormonal stress plus dietary influences may, over many years, promote the evolutionary expansion of a cancerous clone, we still need an exogenous chemical carcinogen to initiate the process if not to drive it. We cannot rule this out but I wonder if we are not over-influenced by the early precedents of environmental carcinogens and, as patients, over-anxious to blame an external villain. Endogenous hormonal stimulation to breast stem cells can itself lead to mutation by at least three mechanisms – accidental errors and misrepair as a consequence of constant proliferation and diminished cell death; direct damage resulting from the endogenous by-products of oxidative metabolism in persistently active breast stem cells; and, thirdly, via a metabolic product of oestradiol itself (hydroxy-oestrone is genotoxic). It's hard to take on board that what seems to be a very normal healthy process can have such deleterious consequences but what is normal in one context can be abnormal in another.

For breast cancer, there is no 'cause' in the straightforward, singular, or usually perceived meaning of the word; no tubercle bacillus equivalent. Neither is a mutant gene *the* common cause. Chronic hormonal stimulation driving persistent epithelial stem cell division seems to be a major factor (cycles driving cycles) and this reflects in large measure our social divorce from evolutionary adaptations for reproduction. But risk is always compounded and in the case of breast cancer, more recent social habits related to diet and energy balance have channelled further risk into the same vulnerable tissues. Superimpose increased susceptibility via genetic inheritance and then add in chance to this prescription and a plausible causal network imbued with evolutionary principles becomes evident.

Even if this causal scenario could be proven to be essentially correct, and formal proof is difficult if not impossible, then there are limits to the conclusions that can or should be drawn. The existence of one predominant aetiological pathway does not preclude others, perhaps in special circumstances, as clearly evidenced from the example of women who have developed breast cancer as a consequence of radiation exposure. Then there will always be patients whose personal, social, and medical history does not appear to fit the preferred or proferred explanation. For those and for any individual patient with breast cancer, the precise causal mechanism will always be elusive. In these circumstances, it is not surprising that patients, their families, and pressure groups feel unhampered in delivering their own verdicts.

In a TV film entitled 'Rachel's daughters: searching for the causes of breast cancer', a group of women shared their very moving personal experiences and conviction that some environmental exposure was responsible for their illness.

Their suspicions are endorsed by the scientists and physicians they chose to interview. The title of the film is a reference to Rachel Carson, famed for her 1962 book *Silent Spring*, the much lauded exposé that alerted the world to wanton pollution of our environment. Rachel Carson herself died of breast cancer at the age of 57 and so the film implicitly suggests that she, as much as anyone, might have appreciated the veracity of the explanation offered by her 'daughters'. They could still be correct in their prescription; it would certainly be a rash scientist who would conclude that environmental chemicals make no significant contribution to the toll of breast cancer. We won't ever know for sure why Rachel Carson developed breast cancer. However, if I had to choose between exposure to an environmental chemical – synthetic, industrial, oestrogenic, or not – and chronic hormonal stress in a woman primed by several million years of evolution for pregnancies but who had none, then I'm sorry but it would be no contest. Either way, breast cancer is almost certainly a preventable illness and there is no greater challenge in contemporary cancer research than cracking this one. And it should be something rather smarter than removing ovaries or breasts, don't you think?

CHAPTER 16

MEN'S TROUBLES

Whilst women have been getting a raw deal from cancer, the tables may now be turning. Cancer of the male prostate gland is fast becoming the most commonly diagnosed cancer in the USA and will overtake lung cancer as a leading cause of mortality in men. And it's out of the closet with the likes of golfer Arnold Palmer and Stormin' Norman Schwarzkopf confronting their own diagnoses on prime time TV. What was previously endured in embarrassed silence is now the talk of boardrooms, golf courses, and the pub.

Current treatments for prostate cancer are crude and provide a sad parallel with breast cancer – surgical prostectomy plus chemical castration with antiandrogens for metastatic disease. The treatment is feminizing and not particularly effective.

In the mid-1990s, around 40 000 males a year in the USA died of prostate cancer and some quarter of a million had a diagnosis of this cancer. This represents a very big jump from two decades before. But therein lies a twist. It has been recognized for several decades that covert tumours of the prostate are common in elderly men dying of other causes. The figures are remarkable. Some 30 per cent of men over 50 years of age have clinically silent prostate cancer and this proportion escalates to over 50 per cent of men over 80. One can backtrack the timing of these lesions by scrutiny of prostate glands taken at autopsy from young men that died of accidents or trauma. In one such study, the first signs of prostatic cancer – low-grade neoplastic lesions (the likely clonal precursor to carcinoma) were detectable in around 10 per cent of men in their 20s. This suggests that the clonal evolution of prostate cancer can be initiated very early, perhaps concomitantly with sexual activity after adolescence, and that the natural history of this cancer is very protracted.

And then, in essence, most men, if they live long enough, develop prostate cancer. For the majority, its potentially lethal consequences will be pre-empted by other more acute causes of death. Much of the apparent increase in the incidence rate of prostate cancer in the USA is due to the instigation of routine examination – rectal tests and serum prostate specific antigen (PSA) testing – which will detect a large number of relatively benign and otherwise invisible cancers. But some of the increase is real, as reflected in both increases in incidence rates in the absence of screening provision (in parts of the UK between 1970 and 1990) and in the mortality statistics, causing widespread concern about its health and economic impact and urgency in identifying its cause. Much of this increase is in middle-aged men (45–65 years) – not just old men staving off other causes of death and thereby providing prostate cancer the time to emerge.

Prostate cancer was considered by surgeons to be very rare before the twentieth century but there are reasons for doubting their judgement on this score. The prostate gland was not identified until the mid-eighteenth century, by the Italian anatomist Giovanni Morgagni, who carefully described the presence of enlarged prostates in men with severe urinating difficulties. It is possible that tumorous growths found associated with the bladder and urethra, not only by Morgagni but much earlier by Hippocrates, were in fact prostate cancers. One of the diagnostic symptoms of an enlarged prostate that may signal either benign growth or cancer – difficulties in passing urine – has been recognized for more than two thousand years as a common ailment of ageing men. But prostate cancer itself was not formally recognized until 1817, when the English surgeon, George Langstaff, described several cases.

So what is the cause of prostate cancer in ageing men? One possible explanation is that it is simply the natural or physiological consequence of living longer. Prostatic senility? Sir Benjamin Brodie, a distinguished surgeon practising in London in the early eighteenth century, thought that prostate cancer was rare but he also held the view that certain pathological changes in the body with age reflected 'that the individual has entered on that downward course, which is to end in his dissolution'. So:

> When the hair becomes grey and scanty, when specks of earthy matter begin to be deposited in the tunics of the arteries, and when a white zone is found at the margin of the cornea, at this same period the prostate gland usually, I might say invariably, becomes increased in size.

Armed with today's diagnostic tools, Brodie might well have identified tumours or cancers in such enlarged glands.

Prostate cancer incidence appears to vary up to fortyfold geographically, from very low levels in some Oriental populations to much higher levels in USA whites and then 50 per cent more in USA blacks. However, these data are at least in part illusory and reflect the screening policies in the USA. Mortality differences are much less – around fourfold. Still, there is some variation in incidence linked to ethnic group which could be either genetic, environmental, or both. Interestingly, clinically covert cancers are as common in Japanese men as in USA whites and blacks. The difference seems to be in the rate of tumour evolution or progression to malignant disease and spread or metastasis. Ethnic

Japanese living in the USA acquire higher rates of prostate cancer than their indigenous counterparts back in Japan (though still lower than other USA ethnic groups).

One school of thought, predominant in the USA, subscribes to the 'find the villain' philosophy. The usual suspects – environmental or occupational toxins, have been rounded up but the incriminatory evidence is at best very weak. Changes in diet provide a more plausible if only partial explanation. Excess calorie intake and unbalanced energy expenditure do appear to be linked to at least a modest increase in risk of prostate cancer. And perhaps when coupled to a deficiency of antioxidants and soy products could explain at least some of the increased risk for Japanese Americans compared with their fellows back home. High levels of the hormone insulin-like growth factor-1 (IGF-1) have been reported to be strongly associated with prostate cancer. If correct, this would suggest a similar explanation to that already offered for diet and breast cancer: more cell division, less cell death (= more cells), more oxidative stress, and more risk to labile DNA. On balance, it seems likely that diet contributes significantly to risk of prostate cancer but other factors must also be involved.

So what else could be going on? Frankly, I don't know the answer and neither does anyone else but I'll offer you a view based upon my prejudice that an evolutionary perspective is likely to be revealing and an irrational desire to see some sort of parity in women's and men's troubles in the cancer business. There are indeed some striking parallels between prostate and breast cancer and both may well be in some way a penalty of the evolutionary imperative for reproductive success.

First of all, the chain of causal events has to involve testosterone (the male hormone). For this the evidence parallels the female breast cancer story with oestrogen. Prostate cancer cells, up until relatively late in their clonal evolution, require male sex hormone (androgens and especially testosterone) for their growth and survival. For this reason, antiandrogen therapy has been the mainstay of therapeutic intervention for several decades. This is exactly equivalent to the oestrogen drive or dependence of breast cancer cells. As you might then expect, castrated males (eunuchs) don't get prostate cancer.

The trouble with testosterone

Let's take a biological look at what the prostate gland is there for. It has evolved in mammals to subserve one, and as far as we know, only one, simple function – lubrication to facilitate sperm flow and fertilization. Its regular function is dependent upon male hormone supply. But then there is an interesting curiosity: the prostate gland in young human adult males is very much bigger than in bulls. In fact, apart from the dog, the human male can boast of a bigger prostate than any other mammal. Somewhat fittingly, the dog is the only other mammal recorded as having an appreciable incidence of prostate cancer with increasing age.

Why should we need such grand prostates? One evolutionary argument comes to mind. Just as at some stage in early hominid development selection for continuous monthly ovulation and covert oestrus or fertility occurred in females, then selective pressure might favour males whose prostate lubrication was at the ready continuously: the primed prostate would clearly be a bonus for a competing male. In other words, we may have been set up again by an evolutionary adaptation that carries in its wake a delayed penalty. A deleterious penalty for the individual but of no impact on his already antecedent reproductive achievements and therefore invisible to the selective forces of evolution. Furthermore, since testosterone levels in men once past 'normal' reproductive age do not decline as severely or consistently as oestrogen levels in females at menopause, then the stimulatory pulses that prime the prostate for activity will continue into an old age when again no selective pressure can operate against any deleterious impact. What was originally an evolutionary advantage now, in another context, imposes a negative trade-off. This seems to me to be a very plausible explanation of why octogenarians of most, if not all, ethnic groups have mini-cancers of the prostate gland.

But we still need an explanation of variable incidence rates of malignant prostate cancer and the probable increases in frequency of malignant conversion in recent decades. Was President Mitterand just unlucky that his prostate got to him before something else? Or was he exposed to some invisible environmental poison that accelerated the growth of a cancer that would otherwise have remained sluggish and benign? Here's a clue. Cancer physicians monitor prostate cancer risk and prostate cancer itself by the PSA test. This laboratory assay detects levels of a prostate-secreted protein in the blood and levels go up considerably when prostate cancer develops. In fact prostate cancer cells also make PSA, providing a potential therapeutic target. PSA levels vary physiologically and rise dramatically, though transiently, in one normal situation – around five hours after sexual intercourse. Now of course this makes sense. If you use up all the lubricant, then in a resilient organ you would expect this to be coupled with a stimulus to replenish supply. Herein could lie the added proliferative and oxidative stress to the prostate that exacerbates an inherent risk of cancer development. Rather than maintain steady production rate of seminal fluid, sexual activity provides regular acute boosts to activity.

Now consider the evolutionary context. What other mammal, including our great ape relatives, continues to indulge in sexual activity long after it can successfully compete with younger, fitter males for the favours of the harem? None of course. The dominant lion or stag or gorilla has his day in the sun, then is outgunned, and dies not long thereafter. Humans, having dramatically uncoupled sex and reproduction, cleverly delay the death trap of most other ageing mammals and carry on, to varying extents, enjoying the fruits of passion. An outlet for their foiled creative fire? And for President Mitterand? His young mistress may have played no role whatsoever in his prostate cancer, but it's a thought isn't it?

So here in a nutshell is a solution to ponder: we have been engineered by long-gone evolutionary events to be the beneficiaries of big, active prostates. The persistent function of the organ over decades and the failure to shut off the testosterone tap on which prostate activity critically depends promotes the inevitable evolution of small or clinically silent prostatic cancer in most men. Sexual activity and unbalanced diets provide the social ratchets that, in concert with sustained testosterone, enhance the risk of these cancers evolving to full malignancy. I know it may be wretched news chaps but that's not the point.

Epidemiological evidence is inconclusive on the possibility that sexual activity might be causally involved in risk, but there are tantalizing hints. Early surveys indicated that simply being married increased a man's risk of prostate cancer but, interestingly, no longer carries this special price tag. Several studies, but not all, have linked prostate cancer with prior increased sexual activity in terms of numbers of partners, frequency of coitus in the ten years prior to cancer diagnosis, a history of venereal disease, or, in one study, desiring more sex than was available. The favoured interpretation of such associations was either that prostate cancer was caused by a sexually transmitted agent (for example, a virus), for which there was, and is, no evidence, or, that sex drive and prostate cancer are two independent consequences of sustained testosterone levels. Sex itself as a promoting activity wasn't considered.

A study of cancer incidence in a cohort of men who smoked marijuana but not cigarettes recorded an increased risk at one site only – the prostate; and at a relatively young age of less than 63 years. This was a small-scale study and needs to be confirmed, but the authors concluded that this highly selective association with cancer type was probably due to the known link between use of psychoactive drugs and sexual activity. In female smokers of marijuana, there was a small increase in risk of one cancer also – of the cervix. Other studies suggested that prostate cancer incidence was less common in celibate Catholic priests than their non-celibate Brothers in other churches. Unfortunately, none of these studies had a large enough sample size and none have asked, or dare ask, the relevant question about actual adherence to celibacy and frequency of orgasms by whatever route. Not that answers to such enquiries would necessarily be believable.

Even if this exotic and speculative explanation for prostate cancer were to hold true, there will as always be more causal contributions to prostate cancer both in general and in specific situations, as there is for breast cancer in women. Prostate cancer has a higher concordance rate in identical twins than any other common cancer which suggests that men vary, genetically speaking, in susceptibility. So what could these inherited genetic factors be? Testosterone levels themselves, governed by an interplay of genetic and environmental factors, are likely to be a major parameter in prostate cancer risk, together with other molecules that play a role in the signal relay between the synthesis of this hormone and its eventual site of impact in the prostate cell.

Variations in testosterone levels in blood appear to be only a weak indicator of prostate cancer risk and are similar in USA whites versus Japanese. But the latter have, on average, constitutively less activity in an enzyme that converts testosterone to its biologically active form, dihydrotestosterone, from which deficit may accrue some protection. In support of this notion, inherited variants of genes that regulate the biological activity of testosterone or its metabolism have been reported to be more common in individuals with advanced or malignant prostate cancer than ethnically and age-matched controls. Next in the firing line is the gene encoding the receptor for dihydro-testosterone on prostate cells – the likely key entry route for proliferative stress and cancer. This varies in its structure between individuals and there is some evidence that a particular genetic variant may be contributing to the above average risk of USA blacks.

Inherited differences, aside from those in the testosterone pathway, will make a difference to risk. Some 10 per cent of prostate cancers occur in the context of a familial incidence and the inherited genes involved in this predisposition will soon be identified. The BRCA-2 gene that strongly predisposes to breast cancer also increases the risk of prostate cancer in families with this particular gene mutation. All told, multiple inherited genetic variations may collectively influence susceptibility to prostate and breast cancer. And then there is chance, as always, hovering in the background. But in the end it all comes back to sex hormones and our entrenched genetic agenda for reproductive success.

CHAPTER 17

CANCER À DEUX

O ver 150 years ago, the French coined the phrase 'cancer à deux' to describe the dual occurrence of cancers of the female cervix and male penis in a cohabiting couple, more often than not husband and wife. How common this was we cannot be sure but it prompted the idea that the cancer might be contagious. It now seems that they were not far off the mark.

Cancers of the uterus have been recognized since antiquity. The Ebers Papyrus (c.1552 BC) gives a remedy for cancer in the womb – fresh dates and limestone pounded with water and injected into the vulva. The writings of Hippocrates (450 BC) also record uterine cancer, although the lack of clear distinction in these and some later descriptions between cancer of the main body or corpus of the uterus versus the cervix does not allow us to gauge the relative frequency of these two very different cancers. Also in the fifth century BC, Hindu texts described surgical procedures for removal of tumours of the cervix and vagina. We can be reasonably confident therefore that cervical cancer has been around for more than 2000 years. More detailed descriptions of cervical cancer began to appear following the rebirth of medicine, surgery, and the arts in the European Renaissance in the sixteenth century. By the nineteenth century, cervical cancer was recognized as a common cancer of women, though those of the uterus, cervix, and corpus were still often pooled together in surgeons' reports.

Cursory observations on lifestyles began to suggest possible causes. Rigoni-Stern, recording cancers in Verona, noted that cancer of the uterus was considerably more common in married women than in unmarried women, including catholic nuns. This led to speculation that either stress or the physical traumas of childbirth was responsible. Other possibilities also began to emerge. The German physician, Adam Elias von Siebold, suggested in 1824 that uterine cancer was due to a scrofulous constitution, venery, and (wait for it) the reading of romances. Von Scazoni in 1861 reported that the cancer was more prevalent in urban women and might therefore be connected with lifestyle. He also ventured the suggestion, without unfortunately providing the evidence, that women with cervical cancer were prone to excessive sexual excitation. Which brings us conveniently if circuitously to the nineteenth-century French observation of an association between cancer of the cervix in women and of the partner's penis. In recent decades, the two cancers have been found significantly associated but the relative rarity of cancer of the penis, which has almost certainly declined substantially in incidence, means that the vast majority of women with cervical cancer will not have a male partner so affected. But the link was and is revealing. Epidemiological evidence is compelling that cervical cancer is associated with sexual activity. As far as women themselves are concerned, risk of this cancer increases with number of sexual partners and is virtually zero in catholic nuns but high in prostitutes. There is also a suggestion that an earlier age of first coupling endows a significant risk, but it is difficult to disentangle this from subsequent promiscuity.

Cervical cancer occurs in all geographic regions but varies considerably in incidence rate. Today it is more common in South East Asia, Africa, and Central and South America. The rate is ten times higher in Spanish-speaking Colombia than in Spain for example. The conundrum is, or rather was, that in some societies with high rates, most women, including those with cervical cancer, were monogamous. Enter what has been called the 'male factor'. Studies in the UK, USA, Latin America, Thailand, and elsewhere have provided incriminating evidence that wayward husbands can be very much involved in causation. There are striking correlations between cervical cancer incidence in monogamous women and the sexual activities of their male spouses. Risk increases up to tenfold for those women married to men who have had multiple extramarital exploits, who frequent brothels, and who, additionally in these situations, eschew the use of condoms. All of which suggests that cervical cancer is in some way an infectious, venereal disease.

In recent years, the finger of suspicion has focused on particular micro-organisms, papilloma viruses. There are more than 100 types of human papilloma viruses (HPVs), several of which are linked to tumour or cancer development. HPV1 and 2 are associated with the common skin wart; HPV6, 10, and 11 with genital warts; and HPV5 and 8 with squamous cell carcinoma of the skin. Papilloma viruses 16 and 18 are now strongly implicated in cervical cancer. Not just cervical cancer but less common cancers of the vulva, vagina, perianal region, and ... penis. So there you have it.

With more sensitive molecular tests, it has been possible to show that over 95 per cent, and possibly all, of the typical cervical squamous carcinomas are infected with HPV16 or 18, although in some parts of the world there are hints that other papilloma viruses are involved. The trends are however worrying. Around 25 per cent of young women in the USA and Western Europe are now infected with HPV16 and HPV18, and there is evidence to suggest that in the absence of regular smear (PAP) tests, we would by now have a real epidemic of malignant cervical cancer on our hands. Precursor tumours are being picked up at an increased frequency in cohorts of women who became sexually active in the late 1960s / early 1970s and it is likely that this in turn reflects changes in sexual activity in girls and in contraceptive practices (that is, the pill replacing the condom).

Given the behavioural conduit for HPV involvement in cervical carcinoma, the antiquity of the disease is not surprising; promiscuity is not exactly a modern trend. The excesses of Caesarean Rome are legendary. Elizabethan London was teeming with hundreds of brothels or 'stews'. It is likely that HPVs were buzzing around in those times but the majority of those most at risk from the long-term cancerous consequences would have died of other more acute causes before a dominant clone emerged from its cervical hide. Still, in all probability, cancer of the cervix is the oldest occupational cancer, for those in the oldest profession.

There is still much to explain. The epidemiological evidence suggests that the interval between likely first infection with HPV and diagnosis is between one and four or even five decades. This very variable and protracted interval or latency can be accommodated within an evolutionary and probabilistic process for cancer clone emergence, although we don't know in this context if the first mutational event prompting cancer clone evolution arises from the initial infection itself or follows later, as a consequence of persistent infection. But then we also need to explain why the majority of women infected with papilloma viruses 16 and 18 don't get cervical cancer.

We know that most young women will clear their infections and many of the early benign clonal lesions regress or remain dormant. Current screening practices also result in the removal of other tumours before they become malignant but, overall, the picture suggests that something else is involved. But then is this really a surprise? Most of us infected with potentially pathogenic viruses, bacteria, and parasites don't suffer any clinical consequences. Credit for restraining the potential of HPVs to provoke cervical cancer must lie in large measure in the immune system. Women who have received transient immunosuppressive therapy are at considerable greater risk (around tenfold) of developing premalignant neoplastic clones in the cervix. Part of the explanation also lies in inherited or genetic factors that influence how the immune system varies between individuals in response to microbial challenges. But more on this in a moment.

Now, following this tale of feminine woe, hands up all those who already knew that cervical cancer was a sexually transmitted disease? Not the majority I guess. Well, there are mitigating circumstances I admit. My *Oxford Medical Dictionary* doesn't list cervical cancer amongst its sexually transmitted diseases. Scientists have suspected for around a hundred years that cervical cancer was in some way transmissible but it's taken until recently to find the agent and illuminate the likely causal pathway. And here again, as in other cancers, a critical causal link has been rendered cryptic by the hidden dynamics of cancer clone emergence and evolution – disguised by both the lack of a simple relationship between exposure (or sexual activity) and cancerous outcome and by the protracted time interval between exposures and a diagnosis. Most other consequences of sexual activity, desirable or otherwise, don't require rare mutational events and slow clonal evolution; their impact is more immediate.

CHAPTER 18

OTHER WAYS OF GETTING BUGGED

Y ou might suppose that cancers caused by common viruses must be very unusual. Not so. Around 15 per cent of the total cancer burden world-wide can be linked to persistent infection with common viruses or other microbial invaders that are transmitted person to person. These cancers are all more common in less developed countries and it is likely that they have been around for a very long time. The links include liver cancer (or hepato-carcinoma) with hepatitis B and C (HBV and HCV); both nasopharyngeal cancer (which is very common in South East Asia) and African Burkitt's lymphoma with Epstein Barr virus (EBV); Kaposi's sarcoma with a new human herpes virus (HHV8); and finally, a form of adult leukaemia (common in southern Japan and the Caribbean basin) that is associated with an RNA virus or retrovirus called HTLV-1. These cancers are all of special interest because of the opportunity they provide for prophylactic vaccination.

The puzzle is that these cancers, like cervical carcinoma, are associated with common viruses with which we have probably cohabited for thousands of years. So why do we appear to be out of equilibrium with them? It clearly doesn't benefit us and what use is it to the virus if the infected host dies? To look at it from the virus' point of view, all it is interested in is making more replicas of itself. Unfortunately for our biology, viral replication exploits the biochemistry of cell replication and does so by inhibiting the proteins that our cells use to restrain proliferation or to induce cell death. Now these are the very same proteins which are critical components of cancers where the genes encoding them become mutated or deleted. That this viral activity can result in cancer is therefore no longer a mystery and, as far as the culprit virus is concerned, it is clearly an accidental by-product of their infectious pursuit of replication. But why do we let the virus get away with it? Isn't this what the immune system has evolved for – to protect us against any harmful effects of common microbial or parasitic infections? And if these viruses can infect anyone, what's so special about the minority (those few per cent) who develop cancer as a long-term consequence? The answers may lie, in part, in the failure of immunological control under particular circumstances.

Most of the cancers mentioned above are characterized by early and persistent infection and a long latency or interval between infection and cancer diagnosis, suggesting a failure of immunological surveillance. In some cases, the basis of this collapse of a normally very efficient protective mechanism is well recognized – co-infection with another virus or parasite which can profoundly suppress the immune system, for example concurrent malaria in Burkitt's lymphoma and AIDS in Kaposi's sarcoma. It's not surprising therefore that when we deliberately use deep immunosuppression clinically to facilitate graft acceptance in transplant patients, that the price to pay is a very much increased risk of some of these cancers – in particular EBV-associated lymphoma, but also HHV-associated skin cancers.

In other cases (HBV with liver cancer, EBV with nasopharyngeal carcinoma, and HTLV-1 with leukaemia) there is evidence that infection very early in life followed by persistent low-level or chronic infection over decades is important in cancer susceptibility. Individuals with persistent HBV infection are some 200 times more likely to develop liver cancer than uninfected persons. This high risk may reflect partial compromise or tolerance of the immune system due to very early exposure with a high viral dose. As a consequence, viruses may acquire the opportunity to chronically usurp normal tissue function and, in their trail, cause cell loss, inflammation, cirrhosis, and ultimately liver cancer.

Genetic variation may play a role, both for the virus and the potential patient. Recent research on papilloma viruses in cervical cancer indicate that uncommon variants or mutant strains of HPV16 and 18 are more frequently present in patients with cervical cancer, implying Darwinian selection of the immunologically invisible. Additional evidence suggests the parental legacy of HLA genes also makes a difference. The HLA genes critically regulate the efficacy of immune recognition and destruction of viruses, and therefore in a confrontation with HPV can tip the balance in favour of microbial knock-out or, by default, the emergence of HPV-driven cell transformation to malignancy.

The likely general interpretation here for viruses and cancer risk rests therefore on arguments about the co-evolution of infectious pathogens and their human hosts, an area of study that Paul Ewald refers to as evolutionary epidemiology. Charles Darwin, in his 1871 *Descent of man*, recognized, before the experimental insights of Pasteur and Koch, that infections were powerful agents for natural selection in 'higher' animals. In the million-year confrontation between microbes and our immune system, there has been selective survival of those individuals whose genetic background, including HLA gene variants, best equips them with an efficacious immune response to particular viruses. But then comes a double whammy. HPV, in common with influenza and HIV, has long adopted the trick of mutating to conceal its identity from the immune system. And, anyway, even if HPV did not have such acrobatic DNA of its own, cancerous or fertility consequences of infection are mostly too delayed or inefficient to give natural selection an opportunity to outflank the microbe.

But clearly low-level persistent infection with these viruses isn't sufficient to cause cancer – it increases risk of malignant conversion. Even in the context of an individual's heightened genetic susceptibility, infection isn't enough; cancer doesn't happen that easily. So what else is needed here? Chance for sure, as with smoking and lung cancer; but maybe other co-factors or modulators of risk as well. Given the social settings or cultural context in which the several common virus-associated cancers occur, then it is also likely, as some epidemiological studies suggest, that malnutrition and dietary insufficiencies may be playing a part in cancer susceptibility. In the case of liver cancers and hepatitis viruses, the answer also appears to lie in part in the presence of other concurrent noxious exposures, in particular, fungal aflatoxins as food contaminants.

Viruses are not the only infectious microbes associated with cancer; animal parasites and bacteria are clearly implicated also. A very rare form of cancer seen in China that arises in the bile ducts has been associated with infection with the fluke parasite *Clonorchis sinensis*. Bladder cancer, in Egypt and some parts of Africa, has been linked with persistent exposure to schistosome (or *Bilharzia*) parasites in contaminated drinking water. We do not fully understand how bladder infection then leads to cancer but chronic inflammation, consequent oxidative stress, and damage to DNA may be important ingredients. A common stomach bacterium, *Helicobacter pylori*, is indicted for gastric lymphoma and is also on trial for playing a part in the more common stomach carcinomas. Chronic or persistent immunological stimulation by the bug appears to promote gastric lymphoma and, rather dramatically, remissions can be induced by antibiotics that kill the bacteria (at least if administered before the cancer has evolved to a highly malignant and independent state).

It is certainly possible that some other cancers, including childhood leukaemia and Hodgkin's disease, have an infectious component to their aetiology. Paul Ewald goes further. In his latest book, '*Plague Time*', he confidently asserts that infections lie at the root cause of most cancers, as well as heart disease and schizophrenia. A bold claim and one, some would say, embarrassingly divorced from supportive evidence.

Whatever the overall toll of infection-associated cancers, it is already recognized to be considerable. And, other than the smoking-related cancers, these are the ones that are most amenable to preventative intervention – by prophylactic vaccination in this instance.

CHAPTER 19

TRAVELLING LIGHT

Each of us is enveloped in a natural coat of skin some one millimetre thick. This layer is continually sloughed off as surely, if less conspicuously, than a snake's and provides a near impermeable barrier of dead and dying cells between our bodies and the outside world. But there is much more to skin than keeping everything in the sausage. It's a complex multifunctional tissue. We have evolved skin for a number of important adaptive reasons – as a barrier to chemical toxins, as a sensory organ, as a social signalling device, and as a heat exchanger.

Skin also protects us from the most ubiquitous DNA-damaging source we are exposed to – ultraviolet (UV) light from the sun. UV light radiates from a part of the sun's electromagnetic spectrum that is invisible to our eyes. UVA, B, and C represent different wavelengths of this radiation. C is almost entirely filtered out by the earth's ozone layer (at least when and where it's intact); B is absorbed by the skin and can directly interact with and mutate DNA (though it is relatively weak compared with UVC). UVA is absorbed differently; it does not damage DNA directly but acts indirectly via the generation of free radicals. The amount of UV exposure humans receive is dependent upon geography (the nearer the equator, the more you get) but also varies with local climatic conditions. The amount of time you spend outdoors and the clothes you wear over your skin will also make an obvious difference to the invisible dose you are receiving.

It's not skin itself that protects us from the DNA-damaging potential of UV light but one particular ingredient – melanin pigmentation, which provides a chemical filter absorbing and scattering UV rays. Melanin is manufactured by a minor population of cells in skin called melanocytes and then distributed in small packets, called melanosomes, to the majority cell type – the skin keratinocytes, as well as to hair follicles and the iris. When hair turns grey, it's because our hair follicle melanocytes have become dormant. Albino traits have inherited mutations in the complex cellular and biochemical pathways that lead to melanin synthesis. Ethnic groups with black skin don't have more melanocytes but produce much more melanin per cell. In particular, they produce a form of brown/black melanin called eumelanin that is a particularly good natural UVB filter. UV filtration efficiency is further enhanced in black skin by distributing melanosomes, diffusely within the keratinocytes. Caucasians make considerably less melanin and in the recipient keratinocyte, the melanosomes are grouped together reducing overall UV absorption capacity. Caucasians that are of very fair complexion make a higher proportion of their melanin as pheomelanin. This yellow and/or red pigment provides a feeble UVB filter and its response to UV light includes the generation of DNA-damaging free oxygen radicals.

Now since skin itself, and its constituent cells and melanin must be made, conveyor belt-like, throughout life, the stem cells lying below the skin surface (or epidermis) are more or less continuously in business, in common with their compatriots in the lung, gastrointestinal tract, and blood. There is therefore an inherent risk of cancer in these cells, particularly since they spend decades in a confrontation with UV light. You might reasonably suppose that melanin in skin is an obvious adaptive trick that allowed us naked apes to set up permanent camp in the tropical sun and as a fortunate bonus provided protection from skin cancer. But it's not quite as simple as that.

But first, a few essential details. Skin cancer comes in three main varieties. Basal cell carcinoma is by far the most common and, fortunately for us, is benign and rarely metastasizes. It usually involves mutations in a gene called 'patched'. This gene has a distinguished evolutionary pedigree befitting its important functional role in cellular development. Very rarely mutated forms of 'patched' are acquired in the germ line and passed onto offspring. This produces the so-called Nevoid basal cell carcinoma (or Gorlin) syndrome for which, as we've already seen, there are some very ancient skeletal imprints. 'Patched' has been around for many millions of years subserving important developmental functions but carrying latent potential to cause trouble.

Squamous cell carcinoma, like basal cell carcinoma, derives from keratino-cytes. It is less common but can metastasize. The third and most deadly variety is melanoma which derives from melanocytes and is highly proficient at metastasis and therefore responsible for three times more deaths than other forms of skin cancer. The incidence rates of melanoma have been steadily increasing since the first reliable data were available in the 1930s, such that current rates are some ten times higher than those of 50 years ago. Some animals such as grey-haired horses and angora goats (in South Africa) develop melanomas as they age but for most animals, melanoma or other skin cancers are rare – unless man intervenes. Expose nocturnal marsupials deliberately and chronically to UV light and they will develop melanoma.

Epidemiological studies have identified risk factors for these skin cancers and although the total picture is incomplete, it is clear that genetic and environ-mental factors interact. Some 10 per cent of skin cancers occur in a familial setting, often as multiple tumours at a relatively young age. Most sporadic or non-familial skin cancers however occur after the age of 50 although, very worryingly, melanoma is now a leading cancer type in young adults. The highest risk is for those with a fair skin and poor tanning ability which places Caucasians, and particularly those of Celtic or Scandinavian stock, in the premier division of risk. Increased numbers of naevi are a harbinger of potential trouble in the melanoma department. Studies of twins reveal that our allocation of these in infancy is under genetic control but most naevi are acquired later, and the increase in number during childhood has been linked to sun exposure. These clonal expansions can be viewed as a useful or adaptive response, but the downside is that in attempting to compensate for their numerical deficiency in pale skin, dividing melanocytes acquire vulnerability as targets for DNA damage if UV exposure is acute.

Black-skinned groups are at a much lower risk of skin cancer. The striking exception of albino Negroids in east Africa provides testament to the protective function of melanin. And when black individuals do get melanoma, it is often on parts of the skin that are less rich in melanin, for example on the palms or soles. A history of intermittent exposure to the sun, coupled with some intense exposure and burning, is a high risk factor for melanoma with total cumulative sun exposure being implicated in the more common squamous cell carcinomas. Living on the north east coast of Australia (Queensland) is perhaps the biggest risk though, significantly, only if you are of Caucasian, colonial stock and not Aborigine.

Although other factors may be involved, there is little or no evidence to implicate tobacco smoking or other chemical carcinogens. Papilloma viruses may be involved in a minority of cases. Transplant patients that have been immunosuppressed have a high incidence of skin warts and are at a greatly increased risk of squamous cell carcinoma of the skin. This reflects viral escape from the immunological jail but since the cancers only occur on sun-exposed parts of the body and are more common in pale-skinned individuals, we suspect that these viruses and UV radiation are co-operating to induce cancer. Skin cancer associated with occupational exposure to oils and tars is a special historical case that we will come to later.

As with many cancers, events relatively early in life can have a substantial impact on later risk. Migrant studies suggest that emigration to Australia from Europe very early in life is associated with acquisition of local high risk rates, whereas with emigration after the age of 18, protection seems to be stamped on the passport. Conversely, high-intensity, intermittent exposure and burning whilst in your teens is very much a harbinger of risk some years or decades ahead.

For many skin cancers, there is convincing evidence that UVB is the directly offending agent. UVB damages DNA in a manner that leaves a unique chemical footprint: a simple but consequential code change in DNA that converts a nucleotide base C (cytosine) type to a T (thymine) type. This presumably occurs throughout the genome of skin cells but as I have explained, will only have adaptive significance or selective value for the potential cancer cell if it fulfils certain criteria. These include when it hits, by accident, a gene whose function is critical for those cells and, also, when the precise position of the mutation, C to T shift in this case, alters the information content of the gene and hence the function of the protein it encodes. These conditions are ably met in basal and squamous cell carcinomas when a large fraction have the C to T signature of UVB in functional hot spots of the *p53* gene.

What's particularly intriguing about this is that we all have mini-clones containing such *p53* mutants. So clearly this is insufficient for cancer clone evolution. One idea is that UVB-induced *p53* mutant clones still form seed-corn for skin cancers to emerge as a rare evolutionary event (risk being in proportion to the number of 'primed' clones). p53 protein plays a major role in inducing cell suicide following DNA damage, functioning as we have seen as a kind of fail-safe device. If it is mutated so as to become inactive, then subsequent exposure to more UVB will allow mutant cells to escape the cell death rule and accumulate more mutations. Additionally, surrounding normal cells, say in burnt skin, will certainly die, and provide space for territorial expansion of the death-resistant *p53* mutants. This seems a very plausible scenario and the puzzling paradox that remains is why all of us fair-skinned individuals don't have skin cancer. The answer must lie not only in the pattern of exposure required (intermittent and intense) but in the rare probability of appropriate genes being mutated in the primed, mutant clone or mini-tumour.

The *p53* gene is seldom mutated in melanoma skin cancer and it is at present unclear what genes provide the functional targets for mutations within the melanocytes. It is also unclear why the melanocyte clone is so precocious at evolving to a highly metastatic state compared with its keratinocyte colleagues. Melanoma cells, as escapees, are the most imperialistic and invasive of the extraterritorial colonizers seen in cancer. I suspect the answer lies at least in part in the prior history of the cell, derived as it is from a highly migratory or invasive stem cell. Perhaps it has retained a genetic memory of this activity and fewer mutations are required to unleash its potential. Another striking feature of melanomas as they evolve *in situ* is the extraordinarily high-density beds of blood microvessels that infiltrate the tumours providing sustenance and potential exit routes. Presumably, melanoma cells are very adept at soliciting this bloody infrastructure support and this may provide them with a major advantage when attempting to set up shop in novel sites outside of the skin.

The evolutionary anomaly

So much for the snapshot description of what happens in skin cancer. The issue here though is how this now very common cancer can be perceived with an evolutionary eye. One obvious point is that the majority of skin cancers develop after normal reproductive age. There is no evolutionary logic for developing or enhancing a protective mechanism that can be effective for two or more decades in excess of what really counts.

That protective mechanisms do exist however seems clear. Not only is this a prime or *the* prime function of melanin but other countermeasures have long been co-opted into work. Since immunosuppressed individuals have a much higher incidence and at a much younger age of squamous cell carcinoma and melanoma, we can assume that the immune response has an important role to play in this type of cancer. Part, and probably only part, of the explanation lies in the association with papilloma viruses to contribute to squamous cell carcinoma development. These viruses are escaping from immune surveillance in immunosuppressed individuals. Another component of the explanation probably lies in the unique ability of UVB to induce, via mutation, novel protein sequences or antigens on skin cells that can be recognized as 'foreign' by the immune system. This may also explain why around 25 per cent of the early clonal lesions of squamous cell carcinoma (called actinic keratoses) regress without treatment.

Another revealing though rare situation is with patients who have the in-herited condition xeroderma pigmentosum. These individuals have inherited mutations in genes responsible for repair of UV-induced DNA damage. It is therefore unsurprising, if depressing, that they have a very high incidence of skin cancers at a young age. Their situation also endorses the importance of protective mechanisms for the recognition and repair of damaged DNA that are of very long-standing evolutionary origin.

But the most striking fact about skin cancer is its association with fair-skinned melanin-deficient humans. Which begs the question of why was emergence out of Africa associated with lack or loss of skin pigment in the first place, at a time when our hairless cousins, staying put, blackened up? That skin pigmentation was an issue at all presumably arose as a consequence of the prior adaptive arrangement to severely reduce the development of body hair. The logic of this dramatic retreat from hirsutism remains a mystery with competing explanations including avoidance of self-ignition around fires and, rather less believably, streamlining for an aquatic existence. We simply don't know the answer to this one, though I'm prepared to give Desmond Morris the last word on this (at least for the time being) since it was he who coined that suitable sobriquet for our species – the 'Naked Ape'. Morris suggested that loss of hair would have facilitated heat loss in a hunter in hot pursuit of prey. However it came about, naked skin was now exposed and we became a variegated species.

The conundrum that invites an evolutionary explanation is why migration and settlement in higher, northerly latitudes some tens of thousands of years ago was associated with pale skin. Whatever the reason is, it is not some genetic quirk of a white-only race of *H. sapiens*. No such thing exists. Caucasians vary dramatically in skin melanin content from very pale (in Scandinavia) to very dark (in Sri Lanka) and the former can move some way towards the latter by scaling up melanin production following UV exposure; that is, tanning.

There have been many competing explanations for the origins of skin of a paler shade. The underlying assumption is that a marked decrease in melanin levels occurred with northerly migration. But surely it is equally anomalous that native inhabitants of Africa have very black skin? Cut off the fur of any primate or mammal and you won't find black skin underneath. Maybe the prototype hairless ape was not particularly dark-skinned (let's say pale brown for the sake of argument) and that subsequent selection for melanin production took different directions depending upon sun exposure, latitude, and other selective forces. Somewhere along the line there was probably advantage to be gained by changing the amount of melanin that our skin normally produces.

There is another, and in a sense trivial, explanation and this relates to what evolutionary biologists call genetic drift. This is applied to a feature that is neutral in its selective value but becomes predominant in a population of humans (or any other species) because that particular group at some time in the past was originally founded by a very small number of individuals or later on passed through a bottleneck in which only a few individuals lived on or reproduced. If one of these reproductively successful individuals just happened to be white or black, then irrelevant as that might be in terms of adaptation, it would eventually become a widespread characteristic in the descended population. Given the multiple genes involved in the control of pigmentation and the striking geographic distribution of skin colour, it seems unlikely that genetic drift is however an adequate explanation of current geographic and ethnic patterns.

This still of course begs the question of why whiter or blacker skin pigmentation should be linked at all to geography. Why then would Aboriginal groups blacken up when staying put in tropical Africa or when colonizing Australasia, especially when this would have retarded heat loss? Alternatively, why stay brown or, more particularly, bleach paler when moving out of Africa?[5] One frequently preferred explanation for the latter puzzle involves vitamin D.[6] This vitamin is required for the absorption of calcium from the intestine for bone growth and maintenance and, in contrast to other essential vitamins, is virtually unavailable in diet. UV light penetrating the skin converts the body's 7-dehydrocholesterol into vitamin D. Daily exposure of an area of skin equivalent to our cheeks is considered to be sufficient for this purpose. Lack of vitamin D produces severe bony abnormalities in the form of rickets. The suggested evolutionary solution is then that at higher latitudes with less sunlight, especially during the winter months, less vitamin D was made in the dark skin, consequent rickets impeded reproductive success, and melanin production was adaptively downgraded, via selection of genetic variants, to compensate for this. Or, to put it another way, rare individuals who just happened, by chance, to have altered the genetic control of melanin production found themselves, rather fortuitously, at a reproductive advantage in more northerly climes. The underlying mechanism would have to be mutation – and, potentially, mutation in any one of very many genes since we already know for mice, and presume for humans, that more than a hundred genes can influence skin colour.

The advantages for the pale faces would have had to outweigh any disadvantages. We can assume therefore that malignant skin cancer was either rare or did not impede reproductive success. But there are some inconsistencies in this explanation. For one, the correlation between skin colour and latitude is variable, though some of the discordance might be accounted for by more recent migration (for example, of Oriental stock into the Americas). Tasmanian Aborigines, as Jared Diamond points out[6], have remained very black. There are other inconsistencies. For example, how come forest dwellers in tropical regions haven't toned down to get more vitamin D? Eskimos living at high, northerly latitudes have relatively dark skin but they may obtain sufficient provision of vitamin D from a diet rich in fish oils – one of the few dietary sources of the vitamin.

Charles Darwin was puzzled by this problem also: 'None of the external differences between the races are of any direct or special service to him'. Darwin's alternative interpretation was that sexual favouritism was at play. Diamond prefers this line of explanation and suggests that if different parts of the globe, for example, Scandinavia, were colonized by small numbers of 'founders' who just happened to have pale skin and for whatever reason found this complexion very appealing in a potential mate, then the trait would rapidly acquire selective currency. Hard to see why Darwin had a problem with this given that this type of explanation – variation begetting selection via reproductive success – is as Darwinian as you can get!

Another way to look at the problem is to recognize that several of the key genes involved in skin pigmentation have other roles in the body including, for example, fat metabolism and blood cell production. It is possible therefore, as

Deol has argued[6], that skin colouration is not strictly adaptive in the evolutionary sense at all. Rather it is an incidental and mostly neutral side-effect of mutations selected for some other conferred benefit that really do have selective value.

As yet we have no clear way to disentangle these different interpretations. In one respect, it doesn't matter. Genetic selection for both pale, melanin-deprived skin and black, melanin-rich skin is a relatively recent evolutionary development, whatever its adaptive significance. And although malignant skin cancer may have an antiquity stretching back two millennia and might even be as old as our species, its incidence rate escalated more recently amongst paler-skinned Caucasians. In the second half of the twentieth century, melanoma tripled in incidence in northern European and USA white males. So what's gone wrong? It is surely the social ratchet at play.

Here, one particular butterfly wing twigging a storm, was the British Government's expedient decision around 200 years ago to banish its minor as well as major criminals to the far shores of sunny Australia, where the highest rates of skin cancer now occur – in vulnerable skins of descendant 'pommies'. The label 'pommie' is used on account of the pomegranate-like red faces the British visitors or immigrants invariably develop when exposed to the subtropical sun. Which leads me on to the second major bad move as far as skin cancer is concerned. This can also be encapsulated in another British phenomenon or phrase – 'mad dogs and Englishmen go out in the mid-day sun' (Noel Coward). Intermittent, intense exposure is delivering the sucker punch especially for malignant melanoma. There are few human social activities that are so blatantly divorced from biology as our tendency to periodically roast our pale, naked bodies in the sun.

It takes no great leap of imagination to identify what behavioural changes over recent decades have brought about this sharp increase in melanoma risk. Personally, as a northerly European, I'll blame it on air travel and cheap package holidays offering easy escape routes from damp and miserably grey climates, increased leisure time, and a vain hope of competing in the mate-catching stakes with those of a more robust complexion. However you look at it, it's a paradoxical measure of our success – in engineering and economics if not in common sense.

But it may be not only in the twentieth century that the pale faces have underestimated the power of the sun's invisible rays. A striking feature of this recent epidemic of melanoma is the relatively young age at which it occurs. The average age of diagnosis is around 50 but many individuals are much younger and melanoma is now the most prevalent cancer in white young men between the ages of 25 and 40 years. So, what about early human migrants re-entering tropical regions? Might it not be expected that Mongoloid groups colonizing the Americas would face problems of UV exposure and skin cancer as they moved south towards the tropics some 15 000 years ago? Mongoloid skin has a protective layer of yellowish keratin that does filter out some UV light but this would have provided insufficient protection closer to the equator. A tantalizing clue may lie in the observation that the skulls, axial skeletons, and skin remnants of several mummified remains of indigenous Inca natives of Peru from around 2400 years ago show characteristic lesions of metastatic melanoma[7] (see Fig. 19.1). If these were indeed melanoma deaths, then it is likely that the incidence of the disease will have far exceeded the current rates in descendant populations in the same regions.

Perhaps the first immigrants to tropical Central and South America, and particularly to the high-altitude Andes in Peru and Bolivia, did suffer a high rate of melanoma. And, in common with many of today's vacationing sun worshippers with melanoma, they may have been relatively young and reproductively active. Obviously this is entirely conjectural but if this did happen, then it follows as a corollary that there might also have been some selection amongst these early colonizers for darker skin and resistance to melanoma. Native Peruvian, Bolivian, and Brazilian peoples do (now) have darker skin colours (albeit not black) than many of their more northerly cousins in the central plains of North America.

Which brings us circuitously back to black. Why did east Africa *H. sapiens*

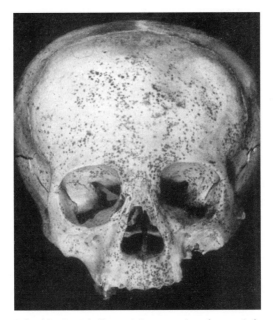

Figure 19.1 Pre-Colombian Inca skull containing metastic melanoma in bone.

blacken up and incur the price of reduced heat loss? One previous explanation, amongst several proferred, that seems credible is that this prevented an *excess* of vitamin D synthesis, from which might have followed calcification of the aorta, renal disease, and premature death. But could melanoma have also been a selective force within the founding Negroid groups colonizing much of Africa or in the descendants of the Aboriginal founders in New Guinea and Australia? Jared Diamond considers that skin cancer would have been a trivial factor in natural selection. But this isn't necessarily so if melanoma rates were relatively high at a reproductive age in relatively small-sized population groups of pioneering founders. Have we always been battling against the sun?

CHAPTER 20

THE GREAT GLUT

An increase in body size combined with a decreased dietary quality leads to a slow moving, fairly sedentary and unsociable ape.

(Katherine Milton, 1993 – with reference to the eating habits of the Hominidae (apes and humans))

I have already touched on the likely impact of diet on cancer risk in the context of particular cancers, but now it is time to give it the 'full monty'. There is an evolutionary perspective on dietary aspects of cancer incidence as well as potential cancer control.

Patterns of food intake and culinary virtuosity vary dramatically between human societies and are part of their richness. The way we eat and what we eat has also changed many times during history, both in recent times and during our evolutionary trajectory from Africa. Along with our great ape cousins, we are derived from herbivorous primate predecessors. But climates change, food sources decline, and we move on. Over millennia, dental and intestinal anatomies will change also, reflecting our nutritional dialogue with nature and the potent selective force that is thus engaged. It is likely that prior to our emergence as erectile species, we shared with other great apes the predilection for plant foods with energy-rich, ripe fruits as haute cuisine. During the oscillating climatic times of the Pleistocene, we came out into the savannah, perhaps in search of food as much as anything else. Meat was then a beneficial supplement to diet, but not a replacement for fruit and fibre. This dietary arrangement is mirrored in current hunter-gatherer tribes. Our ability to tame fire and make weapons and tools will have made a big difference and indeed the need to eat to survive could have oiled the imaginative wheels that spawned these great inventions. Armed with these, we could now adopt plant food sources that would otherwise be too cellulose-rich and indigestible or too replete with toxins. We could catch large, mobile prey and tenderize otherwise tough and unpalatable meat.

From this dietary repertoire came nutritional and other unanticipated benefits. Plant fibre will have decreased intestinal passage time and allowed more consumption of lower-quality foods when richer sources were scarce. A mixed diet of starch-rich plant foods supplemented with meat provided a reasonably adequate source of calories, though most individuals may have struggled to match calorie intake with the energy requirements of a nomadic, foraging lifestyle that was physically demanding, at least episodically.

Plant foods include vitamins and minerals that aid a multitude of physiological processes. And, perhaps as a side-bonus (but one of some consequence) some of these serve as co-factors for DNA repair enzymes and, along with other plant chemicals, especially the flavonoids, exercise antioxidant functions that shut off the major route to DNA damage and mutation. The quality of food has always made a difference to our life, as does quantity.

In our past history, it may have paid to eat to excess and store energy as fat in anticipation that times of plenty would surely be followed by famine – no different in principle to the fattening up of animals preparing to hibernate or migrate. There may even have been some Darwinian selection for individuals equipped with inherited genes whose function enhanced fatty storage (the so-called thrifty genotype). Periodic bingeing would have made some sense.

Our physiology has also been wired up over millions of years of adaptive evolution with circuits of hormonal controls that regulate food intake. Levels of energy input, glucose, and insulin, signal, via the brain stem satiety centre, when it would be prudent to stop or start eating. Eating and its control have always been important. But for most of us the evolutionary and physiological context has been well and truly discarded. Our eating habits are dictated more by pleasure, commercial pressures, and habit than by bodily need, present or anticipated. The ease of access to food, shelter, and entertainment, coupled with revolutionary changes in physical demands of employment have converted post-industrial twentieth-century Westerners into a munching, sedentary variety of H. sapiens. And, much as we would like to believe otherwise, our reaction to food can be as habituated or Pavlovian as a dog's.

Studies of current hunter-gatherer groups provide some insight into the possible nutritional profiles of our Stone Age ancestors. Accepting the caveats that go along with such analyses and analogies, the differences between nutrient and energy sources and energy use now, versus 15 000 years ago, are striking. Our ancestors may have obtained two-thirds of their calorie or energy intake via wild fruit and vegetables and one-third from lean, wild game and fowl, supplemented with eggs and fish. In contrast, the average adult American obtains more than half the average daily intake of calories via cereal, milk products, and nutritionless sweeteners and refined foods. Only 17 per cent now derives from fruit and vegetables. Some 28 per cent of calorie intake is now provided by domesticated meat sources, many of which are rich in polysaturated fats. When these differences are compared with energy expenditure via physical activity, the dietary double whammy is transparent: we now greatly exceed our energy needs whilst having deficient nutrient intake. Skeletal remains of our ancestors throughout the palaeolithic period suggest that we were once tall, lean, muscular, and robust – a physique reflecting a physically demanding lifestyle. Current hunter-gatherer groups are similarly lean.

In Westernized and affluent societies, there has for some time now been an increasing trend to be, in relative terms, big, fat, and physically lazy. Added together these changes conspire to provide us with an excess energy deposit registered as fat or channelled into tissue expansion. More cells, more oxidative metabolism, more nicks in DNA, more trouble? Of course these changes have been coupled with many benefits, but they come at a heavy long-term price to health if overindulged. In biological or evolutionary terms, gluttony and sloth are endemic. It used to be the prerogative of the King of Naples and his ilk but now most of us, in the West at least, have the luxury and temptation of over-indulgence. Nothing like this happens to other less intelligent animals – except that is when we coax pets into some domesticated mimicry.

One-third of Americans and almost as many Western Europeans are clinically obese. And this isn't just the middle-aged and 'oldies' nibbling and napping; some 25 per cent of young American women in their 20s are also obese. News reports will tell you that it's all in your genes and you can't help it. For a minority that may be so but for most, don't you believe it. Your genetics can certainly make a difference (for example, in the ease with which fat is gained or lost) and some people appear to have a decisive advantage in being energy-dissipating fidgets. Some of us just have to try harder than others. This modulator of risk for several major cancer types including breast, prostate, and colon carcinomas, to say nothing of cardiovascular disease and adult-onset diabetes, is important to recognize not least because there is something relatively straightforward we can do about it.

It may seem extraordinary that something as simple as too many calories and too much oxygen-fuelled activity in our cells could be a major factor in cancer risk – but it makes sense. When cancer-prone rats have their calorie intake reduced, their cancer rates decline correspondingly. We are not so very different. But of course that is not all. Our servile adoption of energy-inflated dietary habits divorced from physical needs has been coupled with a decline in the variety and quantity of highly beneficial and protective plant foods consumed. Epidemiological studies to evaluate the impact of diet on cancer risk are notoriously difficult to conduct and confidence in them will also be muted. Moreover, scrutiny of current or recent dietary habits of cancer patients may be an inaccurate indicator of what went on years or decades before when cancerous clones were silently hustling for space. Nevertheless, the evidence from such investigations is persuasive in one particular respect – regular intake of fresh fruit and vegetables does significantly reduce risk of most major cancers. And the link is at least biologically plausible since the evolutionary emergence of a cancerous clone requires oxidative fuelling and DNA damage – processes which antioxidant-rich plant foods can deflate.

Trouble in the back passage

And there is more trouble afoot. Eschewing the vegetables, we greatly reduce our intake of fibre. Our colon and rectum protest; after millennia of facilitating fibrous passage they are entitled to be concerned at the build-up of sludge. The evidence for a link between dietary fibre intake and colo-rectal cancer can be viewed as hard or soft, depending upon your viewpoint. I recall discussing this issue many years ago with the surgeon, Denis Burkitt (of Burkitt's lymphoma fame), who went on to study the changing disease patterns that emerge as Africans became urbanized and 'Westernized'. He was quite convinced of a causal link between diet and colon cancer and bolstered his arguments in a lecture (before dinner as it happened) with pictorial comparisons of excrement size and texture in rural black African versus metropolitan English 'donors'. Burkitt was probably correct in his assertion that the black African increases his risk of cancer of the large intestine by adopting our more refined, fibre-deficient diets, and the association can be biologically rationalized by the simple flushing or purging function of fibre, neutralizing bile acids and other chemical denizens of the gut that might damage the colo-rectal epithelium. Still, epidemiological studies have not been entirely consistent on this score, and it's not surprising. The impact of fibre cannot easily be studied in isolation of the plethora of other dietary effects.

However, there is little doubt that what's on the menu is a cryptic description of the major causal mechanisms at play in colon cancer. Colo-rectal cancer has a roughly tenfold variation, worldwide, in incidence rate. Competition for pole position runs close between USA, Canada, Western Europe, and New Zealand. Men and women within these countries have similar risks and in the USA, there is only a modest variation in risk between blacks, whites, and Japanese (in Hawaii) or Chinese immigrants who have been in the USA for 20 years or more. Rates have escalated dramatically in the second half of the twentieth century for indigenous or native groups that have adopted a Westernized diet and lifestyle (for example, in Canadian Inuits and in Alaskan natives).

Whatever constellation of factors is responsible for colon cancer in the West, it is likely to be very common. And it's not difficult to find suspect dietary themes. Colon cancer worldwide shows a strong association with total red meat intake. The actual biological mechanism at play is not clear however; excess fat used to be the prime suspect but the evidence for this is at best weak. Excess meat could be linked to a dietary deficiency in beneficial plant nutrients and fibre. Lowered risk of colon cancer has been shown to be significantly linked with vegetable consumption. But there is another angle to this story, which brings us back to the gift of Prometheus. There is rather persuasive evidence that consumption of meat that has been subjected to very high temperatures by, for example, chargrilling or frying, is associated with a considerably increased risk of colon cancer. We are back with carcinogenic combustibles, but now being dumped in the intestine rather than sucked into the lungs. Meat proteins subjected to high-temperature pyrolysis (that is, burnt) generate carcinogens, including mutagenic amines, as natural break-down products of organic combustion. Fat dripping from barbecued steaks down onto the charcoal is fired back up onto the meat as a chemical cocktail rich in carcinogenic benzo(a)pyrene and other noxious polycylic hydro-carbons. Another way to smoke? Re-use of frying fat is another sure-fire way of dosing with PCHs. Not the sort of molecules you want to have loitering in any quantity anywhere near your intestinal crypts.

The most likely scenario for the relatively high rates of cancers of the large intestine in the West is a composite of changing dietary habits and cooking modes in silent conjunction with patterns of physical (in)activity. And then studies on identical twins, as with prostate and breast cancer, suggest that some of us are more genetically susceptible to colo-rectal cancers than others.

Salt in the wound?

If the back end of the intestinal tubes take the brunt of this modern dietary assault, at the front end there is a rather different sociobiology and history. Our fast food culture cannot be indicted for everything that's amiss cancer-wise in the guts. Carcinomas of the stomach have been very high in the league table of all cancers throughout the world for a very long time and remain high in certain countries, including Japan and Chile. In the nineteenth century it wasn't only Napoleonic men who developed gastric cancer. It was very com-mon throughout Europe. Virchow had recorded it as the most common cancer in Germany and by 1900, more Americans were dying of cancer of the stomach than any other variety. But, more than any other cancer, this one has declined dramatically in incidence in the West over the twentieth century and by some fivefold in the USA since 1945. That this has occurred in the absence of any deliberate attempts at eradication is fortunate indeed. But what has happened? As far as the original problem is concerned, suspicion focuses on methods used in food preservation and storage and, in particular, the use of salt as a pre-servative and the consumption of pickled and highly-salted foods. Conserving food for future consumption is a useful squirrel-like trait that many animals adopt. Salting or pickling may have been a good idea as well but in acquiring a taste for such foods, we seem to have forgotten that we are not brine shrimps.

Our stomachs are tough but they are not genetically primed for persistent dunking in saline.

Why a high salt content in the stomach should promote cancer isn't entirely clear but it may, in common with and in conjunction with *Helicobacter* bugs, promote inflammation, ulceration, oxidative stress, and, downstream, collateral damage to DNA. Patterns of infection with *Helicobacter* are themselves socio-economic variables. In poor countries, or in economically less privileged sections of wealthy countries, infection is much more likely to occur early in life, setting up perhaps a scenario for persistent or lifelong infection. In parallel with hepatitis B virus infection, this immunological stand-off then permits cancer later on.

The remarkable drop in stomach cancer rates in Europe and the USA may then be due to a fortunate conglomeration of circumstances including the replacement of salty pickling with refrigeration and other means of food preservation plus improving socio-economic circumstances in society and, in particular, better hygiene for infants and children. Changes in human diet, food preservation, and hygiene may therefore, as social variables, have conspired to exacerbate the cancer-promoting capacities of *Helicobacter pylori* over centuries but then paradoxically, and with equally blind benevolence, provided the remedy.

Some like it hot

Further upstream still, there are more socially sculptured disasters afoot. Oesophageal cancers are on the increase in the West, linked in ways that are not yet fully understood, to alcohol intake; the risk escalating in drinkers who also smoke. But elsewhere in the world, there are other patterns of disease that implicate aspects of diet and lifestyle that are long entrenched but still dislocated from those for which our palaeolithic constitution was adapted. In its most striking manifestation, this takes the geographic form of what has been called the 'Central Asian oesophageal cancer belt' (see Fig. 20.1) which cuts a swathe through eastern Turkey, northern Iran and Afghanistan, the republics of Kazakhstan, Uzbekistan, and Turkmenistan, and into north west China (Sinkiang). Women and men appear to be equally at risk of a cancer type that is around one hundred times as common as it is, on average, in Europe. Within the Central Asian belt, there are however sharply demarcated areas of very high and low prevalence of oesophageal cancer. The common link appears to be with Turkic Mongol origin. The high-risk regions correspond to the centre of the old Turkic Kingdom of Uleg Beg and Timur. But it is not, or not predominantly, Mongoloid genes that are important but rather cultural mores that have persisted, little changed, for more than a thousand years.

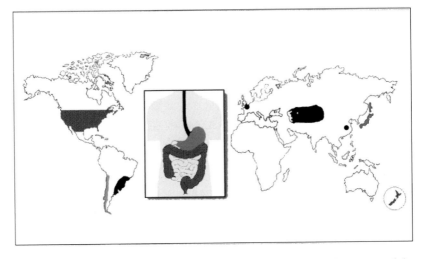

Figure 20.1 World map of intestinal trouble spots, showing high incidence areas of the world for oesophageal, stomach, and colo-rectal cancer.

Evidence for the antiquity of oesophageal cancer in Iran comes from the writings of the Persian physician, Avicenna (980–1037). The list of dietary suspects includes silica fibres in millet, defective trace minerals in soil, and aflaxtoxin mould contamination of stored food. But there are other tantalizing clues to causation and the major chronic assault on the oesophagus probably comes from a unique cocktail of dietary and social customs. Here's the formula: drinking very hot tea, eating the residue from opium pipes, and a staple diet of goat and sheep meat, bread, and cereal but very little of any fresh fruits and vegetables. The link with hot tea has intriguing parallels with the predilection for hot alcohol in the European 'hot spot' for the same cancer (Calvados in France) and with hot maté consumption in southern Brazil, Uruguay, and northern Argentina (the Americas' 'hot spot' for oesophageal cancer). It isn't proven that the link is causal but on the assumption that it may well be, the damage could arise either from the trauma to the oesophageal lining of heat itself or from the ability of hot liquids to provide a solvent for carcinogens.

The other possible risk factor, other than a diet deficient in antioxidants, is an old friend (or foe) in a novel guise. Both in the Transkei in Southern Africa and north-east Iran (high-risk areas for oesophageal cancer) cultural habits of pipe smoking amongst both men and women involve an extraordinary twist. In the Transkei, the tobacco residue in the pipe is either sucked out through a straw and swallowed or scraped out, chewed, and then swallowed. Essentially the same bizarre trait is enjoyed by opium smokers in Iran. These tarry condensates are more carcinogenic, in experimental assays, than cigarette tar, so it seems likely that they are to have a similar, or greater, impact on epithelial cells, albeit diverted into an alternative tube.

Dinner for two

Elsewhere with oesophageal cancer, animal parallels are illuminating. Oesophageal cancer is the second most common cancer in China after stomach carcinoma – though this will be overtaken soon by lung cancer. However, the incidence rates for oesophageal and stomach cancer vary widely and differently within the country. Aside from the Turkic link in north western Sinkiang, there is a separate hot spot for this type of cancer within the province of Honan and, in particular, in Linxian county. Here, the rates for male and female oesophageal cancer are as high as in the Central Asian belt and the lifetime risk of this cancer approaches 10 per cent. And local folklore has it that this has been the case for two thousand years. But the Turkic risk factors do not apply. What does apply isn't known for certain but suspicion falls on a diet that is odd to say the least and may provide another double whammy, in this case of deficient vitamins, minerals, and antioxidants combined with some undesirable additives.

A major component of diet for Linxian peasants is pickled vegetables which, strictly speaking, are not pickled but boiled and stored in jugs for around six months, by which time the vegetable mulch has a coat of fungal mould. The whole mouldy mash is eaten and is said, by Westerners at least, to smell like silage. Epidemiological studies in Linxian have so far failed to establish a clear link between consumption of mould-ridden vegetables and oesophageal cancer. It is known however that these moulds are a rich source of carcinogenic nitrosamines, and other studies have linked pickled vegetable intake with chronic oesophagitis (in 15–26-year-olds in Huixian province) and with oesophageal cancer itself, in Hong Kong Chinese.

A further clue comes from the chickens the peasants keep. They are regularly invited to partake of the same mouldy concoction and it seems a remarkable coincidence - if it's a coincidence at all – that they appear to have a high rate of an equivalent cancer (of the gullet). It may also be relevant that the chickens are kept until what is, for them, an old age; the majority of gullet cancers were in chickens that were more than five years old. Further indictment of the mouldy vegetable comes from the following anecdote. Following the building of a large dam and reservoir, some 50 000 peasants from Linxian were moved to another province, Hubei. They took their diets and their oesophageal cancer risk with them but left their chickens behind. Once ensconced in their new abodes however they, naturally enough, acquired local chickens. A subsequent study of many thousands of chickens revealed cases of gullet cancer in some of the 'adopted' chickens but in none of those residing with the native inhabitants. Not unambiguous evidence maybe, but if I was a chicken, I would ask for a transfer.

Meanwhile, Chinese scientists, in collaboration with the US National Cancer Institute, have conducted a unique nutritional intervention trial in Linxian. From 1985, some 30 000 adults (40–69 years old) were provided with dietary supplements of specific vitamins and minerals in one of four different combinations. Cancer rates were then assessed over the following five years (a short interval in the context of the evolutionary trajectory of cancer clones). There was evidence for a reduction in stomach cancer for those receiving daily supplements of beta carotene, vitamin E, and selenium and a suggestion of a reduction in oesophageal cancer in those given riboflavin and niacin. The Chinese authorities have also put in place a massive public education and early detection/screening programme in Linxian. Consumption of 'pickled' vegetables has been discouraged and new storage methods reducing mould contamination introduced. There are indications that mortality rates are now declining. If this holds up, it will provide a truly remarkable example and important precedent for cancer prevention.

One other animal parallel is with oesophageal cancers in Scottish cattle. Here, certain papilloma viruses are identified as causative agents but work in silent conjunction with immunosuppressive and carcinogenic chemicals that occur in the bracken ferns on which these animals graze. In the one human population that, bizarrely, finds bracken palatable (the Japanese) there is a similar association between consumption and increased risk of oesophageal cancer.

Clearly for many of the very distinct and geographically disparate cancers that are associated in some way with diet, we have no robust evidence identifying exactly what combination of factors are critical in causation. But there is little doubt that idiosyncratic and social aspects of our acquired dietary habits for which we are genetically ill-adapted are at the root of it. If the impact were acute or poisonous then, as with any other species, exploring dietary options, natural selection, or aversion behaviour would have been the natural remedy. Cancer, unfortunately, is a chronic ailment; it works its way through, inefficiently and at a snail's pace, over decades. It would be a mistake, however, to carry on regardless in anticipation that epidemiologists will deliver black and white answers on something as complex as diet or that biotechnology will provide the cure-all pill.

CHAPTER 21

DYING FOR A LIVING

Some argue that bacteria or insects are planet Earth's most successful life-forms. In terms of persistence, sheer numbers of individuals or species, and extraordinary environmental adaptations, they may well be. Mosquitoes usually get the better of me. But even a cursory observer from another planet would surely single out *Homo sapiens* as rather special. We are an extraordinarily dextrous and inventive species. We are enterprising at making things; superb at construction and destruction – and on a massive scale. In so doing we have drastically altered our habitat and can generate quite novel environments – no more so than where we work. Working for a living, as everyone knows, can seriously damage your health. Workers down the ages have been burnt, poisoned, drowned, or squashed, or have died of sheer exhaustion.

Bernardino Ramazzini's famous quote about nuns and breast cancer (see page 139) was part of a remarkable treatise or 'Diatriba' on illnesses associated with different professions. First published in 1700, *De morbis artificum*, or *Diseases of workers*, is an epidemiological landmark, linking for the first time preponderance of certain illnesses with indecent exposures in the workplace. Although much of his evidence appears anecdotal or second-hand, his views on the diseases of miners, cleaners of cesspits, vintners, corpse bearers. and 'learned' men makes interesting and entertaining reading. But the dangers were, and are still, in most cases, up front to be seen or sniffed, with any deleterious impact not far behind. With the altogether more insidious cancer, it has been very much delayed payment.

Industrial, commercial, or medical enterprises can involve concoctions of uniquely high local concentrations of mutagenic substances. Many of these chemical or radioactive insults are natural substances – derivatives of or synthetic copies of natural substances which normally exist in our environment at easily tolerable doses. But the tissues, cells, and DNA of individuals exposed to high concentrations face an unnatural and unanticipated challenge that can outflank the efficacy of our rich evolutionary adaptations for survival. Cancer can be one consequence of acute or chronic occupational exposure.

The first epidemic

Percival Potts' recognition, in the eighteenth century, of scrotal skin cancer in chimney sweeps, is usually portrayed as the first example of an occupational cancer. It's an instructive tale but it has an important precedent. Historically, the oldest known industrial or occupational cancer is in fact lung cancer. Ironically, perhaps, this has nothing to do with fire and cigarettes and involves an entirely natural substance – radon. Radon gas is a natural radioactive product of uranium and is a constituent of many common geological formations, such as granite. Normally this gaseous product would seep slowly into crevices and to the surface, but mining can stoke up abnormal clouds of activity. Inhalation of radon or of dust particles coated with radon or its radioactive breakdown products (or 'daughters') including polonium, can irradiate the lung and mutate DNA.

Mining for tin, fluorspar, iron, and especially uranium, have all been associated with increased risk of lung cancer. Mining for uranium for military purposes began in the 1940s in the Belgian Congo (Zaire), North America, East Germany, and, later, in France. Little or no appreciation of risk from gaseous radon exposure existed and protection afforded to workers was minimal. Studies in the USA during the 1950s and 1960s established a link between radon exposure and excess lung cancer that was in fact greater than the excess of all cancers in survivors of the atomic bombs in Nagasaki and Hiroshima. Many of the dead were Navaho Indians employed in the uranium mines of New Mexico. This startling discovery was subject to political embargo but did eventually lead to the belated introduction of monitoring devices, ventilation, and better worker protection. Much of the damage was by then done however.

It has been estimated that some 250 000 miners worked underground in the 1940s and 1950s in the East German uranium mines, and perhaps as many as half a million worldwide. The East German mines under the postwar control of the Soviets were concentrated in the region of Schneeberg which lies on the northern slopes of the Erzgebirge or Ore mountains. Previously secret medical records of almost half a million uranium mine workers came to light after the fall of communism and revealed that thousands had either died or were, at the time of recording, suffering from lung diseases including silicosis and lung cancer.

Extraordinary and unique as this disaster might seem, it has a remarkable historical echo in the Ore mountains. Mines in both Schneeberg and in Jachymov (on the southern slopes of the Ore mountains) were dug extensively for silver as long ago as 1470, and already by the early sixteenth century, it was recognized that the miners were unusually prone to lung diseases, referred to collectively as 'Bergsüchte' (and later called Schneeberg Lung Disease). The frequency of disease appeared to increase in the seventeenth and eighteenth centuries when mining not only for silver but for copper and cobalt was stepped up. The predominant lung disease was eventually recognized as lung cancer in the 1870s by two local physicians, Hesse and Härting, who calculated that 75 per cent of former miners died from the disease. Its cause remained unclear however; inhalation of various metals in ore dust being suspected.

Somewhat symbolically, it was from the Jachymov mines that Marie Curie and her husband first obtained radioactive radium (which decays to radon gas) and polonium (from pitchblende). Conditions in the mines continued to be atrocious even after radon levels were measured and shown to be extremely high. In reviewing this sorry tale of ignorance, neglect, and exploitation, Jacobi points out that the mine with the highest measured radon concentration was known to the workers as 'Todesschacht' or the 'death mine'.

By 1913, H E Muller, working for the miners' social community, concluded that Schneeberg lung cancer was an occupational disease attributable to radium emissions in the mines. But this view was not generally accepted by most medical scientists involved who entertained alternative causal mechanisms, including dust inhalation and pneumoconiosis. Sadly, it was to take another two decades before, in 1940, extensive studies led by B Rajansky finally provided firm evidence that radon inhalation was almost certainly the cause of the great excess of lung cancers. And then, in 1946, along came the Soviets and their East German buddies who promptly ignored safety recommendations. The Soviets were desperate for uranium to develop their atomic bomb. No bomb was dropped but it is estimated that around 10 000 to 15 000 miners in total will have died unnecessarily of lung cancer in the wake of this military agenda. In this respect, the Soviets and USA governments were equally culpable.

More pyrotechnics, warts and all

But arguably the most important historical examples of occupational cancer bring us back again to fires and carboniferous combustion. Skin warts, leading after many years to cancer of the skin (frequently on the scrotum), have been an occupational hazard for men engaged in seemingly quite different professions, including chimney sweeps and workers plying a variety of trades in which they were either producing or using tars and oils. What they have in common is chronic exposure of the skin to carcinogenic or tarry products of partial combustion – and the same delayed, cancerous consequence. The causal route to these cancers has an extended history.

Freshly hewn wood or its partly burnt counterpart (charcoal) has been used in fires for millennia. This combustible fuel source produces only a modest level of smoky products and residual tar. The colonial Romans, in Britain, were perhaps the first to recognize the fiery promise of fossilized organic coal and to mine it for this purpose. The first mining of coal under commercial licence was in 832 in Britain but it was not until the fourteenth century that coal came into more general use. Burning coal generates, along with heat, a considerable amount of smoke which made it socially unacceptable for a long time. During the Elizabethan period in London, coal fires could not be lit when Parliament was in session. A number of interrelated events during the sixteenth and seventeenth centuries changed this situation. In essence, fuel demand escalated as wood sources became scarcer and more expensive. Fuel was required not only for heating homes but for new industrial processes such as glass manufacture, brewing, and dyeing. Coal came to usurp wood as the natural carboniferous source of heat.

Accidental fires spreading outside the confines of the hearth (or mouth) have provoked collateral damage ever since the talent for ignition was invented. The Great Fire of London in 1666 was a landmark in this respect. During the preceding century, brick and stone had begun to replace wood as building materials. Most houses then had internal fires and some sort of chimney for the conveyance of smoke. One outcome of the Great Fire was that longer chimneys became very common. But then they were prone to clogging up with soot: the chimney sweep trade took an upturn.[8]

> To look like her are chimney sweepers black.
>
> *(William Shakespeare, Love's Labours Lost, Act IV, Scene III)*

Sweeps had been plying their trade during Shakespeare's time and for at least a hundred years before the Great Fire. After London's burning, sweeps increasingly used small boys as young as five or six to assist by climbing up into the narrow flues. Apprenticeship carried its reward of lifelong employment, and its penalties of pulmonary disorders, dermatitis, warty skin growths (known in the trade as soot wart), and, after many decades, skin cancer. The link with skin cancer and, in particular, cancer of scrotal skin, was first recorded by Sir Percival Potts, surgeon of St Bartholomew's Hospital in London, in 1775. He suggested the prior practice of regarding the disease as venereal and best treated by mercurials was ill-advised and that the only chance of 'preventing the mischief' was to extricate the lesions quickly before the cancer spread throughout the testicle then to the local lymph nodes and abdomen. Potts' patients were relatively young compared with most of those with cancer that he saw and he clearly had a great deal of sympathy with their plight; hence Sir Percy's lament:

The fate of these people seems singularly hard; in their early infancy, they are most frequently treated with great brutality, and almost starved with cold and hunger; they are thrust up narrow, and sometimes hot, chimnies, where they are bruised, burned and almost suffocated; and when they get to puberty, become perculiarly liable to a most noisome, painful, and fatal disease.

(Sir Percival Potts, 1775)

And so it continued for a long time. All told, scrotal skin cancer from soot exposure has a track record in England of around 300 years.[8]

Some perceptive professional observers of the cancer scene in the nineteenth century conjectured that the mechanism of cancer causation by soot, and even the offending but invisible chemical(s) involved, might parallel the cause of oral cancers and tobacco smoking. Soot, as a residue of carboniferous combustion, does contain some of the same obnoxious molecules as cigarette tar, including benzo(a)pyrene, but the chemical cocktail is different and its major offensive carcinogen is probably another polycyclic hydrocarbon called cyclopenta(c,d)pyrene.

But then comes a puzzle. In the nineteenth century, sweeps' cancer was generally recognized in England by both surgeons and sweep journeymen themselves as a token of the trade. But at the same time it was evident that scrotal cancer was exceedingly rare amongst men plying the same business in countries of continental Europe and the USA. Sir Henry Butlin, Professor of Pathology in Surgery at the same London hospital as Percival Potts (St Bartholomew's), sent his assistants trudging round the fire stacks of Europe to find the answer to the English disease. What was quickly apparent was that the sweeps of Germany, as might have been anticipated, were much better organized; they wore more protective clothing and washed more thoroughly and more regularly. And they looked pretty cool dudes too (see Fig. 21.1). The same applied to the sweeps in Holland and Belgium – with respect to their prophylactic habits that is. The French were a problem though. They were as soot-laden and ill-equipped as their English counterparts. So was it their toiletry that saved them from the dreaded wart? Butlin thought it unlikely:

For, seeing that the dress worn by Paris sweeps ... does not protect the body from the contact of soot, the active absence of the disease would auger a degree of personal cleanliness on the part of the men which is wholly inconceivable to any person who is acquainted with the general habits of the French lower classes in that respect.

Voilà!

The other variables that impacted considerably on risk were, Butlin suggested, the type of fossil fuel used, the structure or openness of the fireplace and stack, and the amount of soot that would be generated by these. His

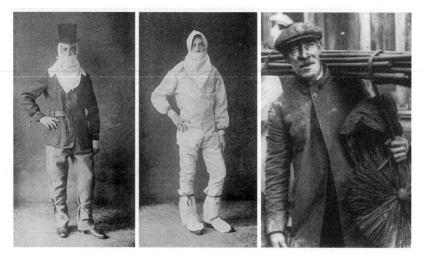

Figure 21.1 European sweepstake. Left, German sweep *c.* 1880; middle, Belgian sweep *c.* 1880; and right, English sweep *c.* 1930.

European sortie and survey may have been somewhat cursory but it was evident that whilst England used so-called hard coal for fires, other countries, where sweeps' scrotal cancer was rare, more often used wood, coke, and charcoal, all of which generate far less sooty residue.

This fire, soot, and warts tale is instructive in the general context of causal networks in cancer. The essential and proximal cause or offending agents we now know are the chemical carcinogens in combustion products in soot to which sweeps can have a substantial and chronic exposure. But the actual risk of cancer is heavily modulated by other social and technical variables including, in this case, choice of fossil fuel and, especially, relatively simple aspects of clothing and cleanliness. On this basis, Butlin suggested, preventing this cancer was, in principle, straightforward.

Some 100 years after Potts' report, medical evidence began to emerge linking skin warts and cancers, including scrotal skin cancer, with occupational exposure to shale oils, pitch, and tar. When, later in 1922, Drs Southam and Wilson reviewed the occupations of 141 men that had been diagnosed with cancer of the scrotum skin at the Royal Infirmary in Manchester over the previous 20 years, they were surprised to find that only one was a chimney sweep. Twenty-two were tar and paraffin oil workers, which was not entirely unexpected, but 69 were men working the spinning machines or mules in the Lancashire cotton industry. Mule spinners also had a high incidence of dermatitis and skin warts. The majority of these patients with scrotal cancer had worked on the mules for most of their working lives and their cancer usually had a well-defined scrotal wart or mini-tumour as an antecedent. A lethal outcome evolved from a benign beginning.

Operating the mules was an exclusively male activity. In the nineteenth century, boys started this work at the age of eight to ten years. One patient diagnosed with scrotal cancer at age 75 had started work on the mules aged six, in 1866. For most, the data suggests a very long interval of several decades between first exposure and progression to cancer, the average age of diagnosis being in the 50s. From census data, it was calculated that for the 23 000 men who were employed in this task, the risk of dying of scrotal cancer was around 1 in 2000 each year. By way of comparison, Archibald Leitch calculated that in the 1920s the risk of a chimney sweep dying of scrotal skin cancer was around 1 in 1400 each year.

Leitch also suggested a plausible solution to an anomaly with scrotal cancer. Since sweeps in the eighteenth century, the early twentieth century, and even in my own youth were habitually covered in soot and mule spinners' skin was similarly exposed to the hot shale or paraffin oils that lubricated the moving parts of the mules, why was the scrotum the hot spot for cancer? Leitch conjectured that warmth was part of the answer, combined with the solvent properties of the sebaceous secretions of the scrotum. But there was another anomaly to resolve; a rerun of the Henry Butlin enquiry took place. Workers in Germany and the USA similarly exposed to shale oils and tars, for example in paraffin manufacture, had a considerably lower incidence of scrotal or skin cancer than their English counterparts. Other contributory factors that increased risk for the Lancashire mule spinners included the quantity of unrefined oil used on their mules and to which they were exposed and the lack of provision of any washing facilities – that and standing close to an oil-covered movable shaft or carriage. Southam and Wilson, as part of their epidemiological detective work, visited the factories and noticed that the men, lightly clad in a hot moist environment in cotton trousers or overalls, usually had a well-marked oil zone between their upper thighs and abdomen where they persistently leant against the oiled carriage of the mule.

Tars and paraffin oils had been recognized as a likely source of carcinogens and causal agents for cancer of the skin in exposed workers since 1875 in Germany and these observations were very instrumental in opening up a crucial era of cancer research. Rabbit skin painted with tars developed similar warts and tumours and provided a bioassay for the purification and identification of chemical carcinogens in tar. Chemical carcinogens in mineral oils were therefore the offending agents but very much aided and abetted by poor working conditions – that and chance.

The identification of cancers due to occupational exposure to soot, tars, and oils had a major impact on the public perception of cancer and on cancer research. By 1907, scrotal cancer was added to the Workman's Compensation Act, the definition being 'scrotal epithelioma occurring in chimney sweeps and epitheliomatous cancer or ulceration of the skin occurring in the handling or use of pitch, tar and tarry compounds'. But there was a catch. In order to be considered for compensation, the cancer had to be diagnosed whilst still employed or no later than 12 months of ceasing to be a worker in the relevant occupation. Older age cancer didn't count and no compensation was ever available for workers whose scrotal skin cancer finally evolved to full malignancy 1 to 35 years after retirement. Nevertheless, it was a mule spinner with scrotal skin cancer that provides the first example of litigation against an employer for cancer due to occupational exposure. The plaintiff won. Moreover, in 1920, skin cancers became notifiable diseases under the Factories Act, which meant that incidence rates could be documented and preventive measures introduced and monitored.

Sundry poisonous profits

The International Agency for Research on Cancer (a WHO-associated organization) takes a major responsibility for scrutinizing the evidence for carcinogenic substances. They have classified more than 40 hazardous industrial or workplace exposures as being associated with an increase in specific types of cancer, most of which could have been avoided with relatively simple and inexpensive improvements in working conditions. The most notorious involves asbestos. These natural silicate fibres have been recognized for centuries for their fire-resistant, heat-retaining properties. Inhalation of asbestos fibres is unequivocally associated with a normally exceptionally rare but very malignant type of cancer of the pleural linings of the lung and peritoneum (mesothelioma). The lifetime risk for those most exposed is extraordinarily high and even modest or very transient exposure appears to be risky – more so than tobacco smoking, perhaps because the fibres, once inhaled, persist.

The biological mechanism of carcinogenesis is less clear than with tobacco but probably involves chronic inflammation, oxidative stress, and consequent 'accidental' mutations in cells. The emergent history of the link between asbestos fibres and lung cancer runs remarkably parallel to that of the tobacco saga. As Robert Proctor has vividly recorded, the industrial profiteers used the same tactics of denial, obfuscation, and deceit to protect their trade long after the hazard was recognized.

Chemicals including benzene, vinyl chloride, and 2-napthylamine and other aromatic amines used, in the past, in the rubber and dye industries, have all been linked convincingly to cancer. In total it has been calculated that some 200 000 past deaths in the USA are attributable to occupational exposures. The figure could be higher. Safety legislation has belatedly reduced hazardous occupational exposures in most developed countries but no such protection is afforded to many workers in the majority of underdeveloped but neo-industrialized third world countries. Here the cancerous hazards remain and are probably increasing. At the same time, multinational companies responsible for propagating this route to profit hide their ethical and legal responsibilities behind local subsidiaries. The same applies to the purveyors of cigarettes. It's in the developing nations that the cancer burden will increase most in a grotesque reprise of our oncological history – but on a larger scale.

And back home? Current risk estimates of cancer from industrial exposures in the West have been highly contentious and fears easily exacerbated by striking anecdotes, bad track records, secrecy, suspicion, and embellished to some extent by political and ideological motives. Given the now revealed industrial track record, some scepticism is not only inevitable but desirable. Continued vigilance, safety legislation and monitoring, and some prohibition are certainly called for. Still, some staunch advocates of the 'industry is the villain' thesis for cancer continue to exaggerate the risk contribution from this source and unfortunately in so doing, compromise the credibility of the important issue they wish to address. Epidemiologists Doll and Peto calculate that no more than 5 per cent of the total adult cancer burden in the USA can be so ascribed. Even if correct, this still translates to a far from trivial number of cancer deaths (around 25 000 per year in the USA alone), especially as much of the risk and cancerous potential is not evenly spread but is likely to come from point sources, some invisible, and over which those exposed have no control. We are not entirely out of the woods in respect of this risk.

CHAPTER 22

COLLATERAL DAMAGE

T he final causal pathways for cancer to consider are those that have arisen uniquely in the twentieth century, and as a by-product of our extraordinary technical virtuosity. These are all relatively infrequent but instructive examples of delayed and collateral damage where initial intentions were either benevolent or malign.

Hit by friendly fire

Many medical treatments, including radiotherapy and chemotherapy, are effective because they damage DNA and kill cells. Inevitably then, patients are subject to a double jeopardy that can, occasionally, lead to the most ironic of outcomes: cancer caused by cancer therapy itself. Or, to recall a phrase from the Gulf War that is as memorable as it was awful – hit by friendly fire. Historically, this is akin to inadvertent poisoning from arsenic or other remedies considered to be beneficial for medical conditions.

The collateral damage and its consequences arise because radiation and many medicinal drugs lack specificity. A small percentage (around 1–5 per cent) of patients with leukaemia, Hodgkin's disease, ovarian, and other cancers have developed so-called 'secondary' leukaemias or, less often, other cancers that can be attributed to their prior therapeutic exposures. One of the more tragic and dramatic examples of this is the very high accumulated or overall risk of breast cancer in women who received broad-field chest X-rays for Hodgkin's disease when they were aged between 13 and 16 years. The figure is around 40 per cent or 4 in every 10 exposed. Most of these women will have developed breast cancer 20 to 30 years after the initial mutational event. That the risk was particularly high for such young women, but less for older women, probably reflects the hormonal physiology of the breast in the post-pubertal period when stem cell proliferation may be high and therefore risk from DNA damage correspondingly increased. Procedures for therapeutic irradiation have now changed with the introduction of shielding and more focused beams, so this risk has been much reduced.

A historical precedent for X-irradiation-induced cancer lies, ironically, with those physicists, chemists, and doctors who first harnessed natural radiation for our benefit. Marie Curie and her daughter Irene both died of radiation-induced bone marrow failure. Marie Curie herself was so hot that her letters remain radioactive to this day. Leukaemia incidence was considerably increased in the early hospital radiographers using poorly shielded apparatus. This particular problem was recognized and dealt with in the Western world but persisted unchecked in some countries such as China well into the second half of the twentieth century. By 1902, just seven years after Röntgen's discovery of X-rays, it became clear that exposure caused not only painful erythema and dermatitis but, in some individuals, malignant skin cancer, usually on the hands, and within a relatively short period (a few years). A quarter of a century later, there was a strong clue to its mechanism when H J Muller discovered that X-rays caused mutations in the *Drosophila* fruit fly. But the significance of this observation for cancer causation was missed at the time. This was not without consequence.

The widespread vogue for therapeutic and diagnostic use of radiation during the 1930s to 1950s did not appear to have been accompanied by an appreciation of the likely risk involved. In the cohorts medically exposed for ankylosing spondylitis, benign gynaecological conditions, or even scalp ringworm, there was a consequent excess of leukaemias. And for women with tuberculosis having fluoroscopy examinations – a delayed double whammy of breast cancer. In the same period, there was an increase in risk of around 40 per cent for childhood leukaemia following use of X-rays for diagnostic pelvimetry in pregnancy. The use of ionizing radiation for diagnostic purposes has changed very markedly since that time and there is no evidence that current practices (dental X-rays for example) carry any risk.

Another tragic example of therapy begetting cancer is the relatively high frequency of lymphomas as well as some skin cancers and cervical carcinomas in patients receiving immunosuppressive therapy – either as kidney or heart transplant recipients or for autoimmune diseases. In these instances, the greatly increased risk arises primarily as the consequence of common herpes or papilloma viruses being let off the immunological leash that normally restrains their capacity to promote the development of cancer. Skin cancer developing as a unintentional consequence of treating psoriasis with UV light plus photo-activated compounds (psaloran) is another telling, if sad, illustration of the collateral damage route to cancer.

One response to this gloomy litany of cancers inadvertently facilitated by doctors is to question how far we have drifted in our approach to the treatment of disease. So-called 'secondary' cancers are but one aspect of the undesirable downside or morbidity associated with blunt or non-specific therapies. There is a case to be considered here in the context of current cancer therapy as we will see later, but cynicism is out of order. Physicians have to make do with the best of what is available, often in crisis situations. Inherently toxic and dangerous therapies are used on the basis of a risk–benefit calculation. The reasonable argument used is that an increased risk of cancer or other morbid side-effects arising from treatment that may be curative or prolong life for a patient with an acute and otherwise incurable illness is usually preferable to the stark alternative. But the prospect for a pyrrhic victory must loom large in the calculations and the assumption must be that the patients themselves are fully informed and understand the equation.

Or by decidedly unfriendly fire

Many microbes, animal species, and even a few plants are belligerent but *Homo sapiens* is unique in the extent to which he uses his technical prowess to exterminate members of his own species. Extraordinary ingenuity has been employed in order to bring about the demise of a perceived enemy or rival. The spear or the bullet can provide a quick if traumatic exit. Other assaults are somewhat slower, no less lethal, and certainly more painful. Mustard gas used extensively in the First World War and in the more recent Iraq–Iran skirmishes is a lethal chemical. Its toxicity to the skin, lung, and particularly bone marrow can kill relatively quickly. It is also a very powerful chemical carcinogen that mutates DNA. It is highly likely that many exposed soldiers and civilians who received sublethal exposures have gone on to develop cancer but no follow up of these unfortunate victims has ever taken place. It's also one of the ironies of the cancer story that the potency of mustard gas in damaging DNA later gave rise to two of the more effective genotoxic agents used in cancer chemotherapy – melphalan and chlorambucil.

But the pinnacle of man's application of his creative skills to belligerence was reached in 1945 when the two nuclear bombs were dropped on Hiroshima and Nagasaki. Many were killed in the initial explosion and hot blast, others died in the short aftermath of acute irradiation sickness. For others some distance (about 1500 metres or so) from the epicentres, there was a delayed legacy of cancer. The atomic bombs remain the most potent point source, in time and space, of an engineered cancerous insult. In the years that followed the explosions, there was a marked increase in leukaemias in particular, of thyroid cancer, and a more modest but still significant rise in breast and some other cancers in the exposed population. Risk was directly proportional to dose received or proximity to the epicentre. So much so that the Japanese risk associations for cancer monitored in over 100 000 survivors, by the so-called Life Span Study, have provided the benchmark for calculating potential risk from much lower-level chronic exposures and for legislation in setting safety standards. The acute or single dose of gamma irradiation received by those who developed leukaemia was estimated, in units called Grays, to be from 1 to 4. This is approximately the same as some therapeutic doses in medicine but around 1000 times our natural environmental exposure level per year. A total body exposure to 5 Grays is usually lethal. It is not at all surprising then that this exposure was a causative agent for cancer. What is perhaps more surprising is that the great majority of those exposed at this level did not get cancer. It is likely that they all incurred mutations in DNA; indeed these can be demonstrated today in healthy survivors' blood.

As with therapeutic insults and other carcinogenic exposures, chance plays its ubiquitous role. It will have been a lottery in Hiroshima and Nagasaki whether gamma emissions ionized and irreversibly damaged a cancer-relevant gene in a cancer-relevant cell that survived the insult. Even with the most vociferous of insults, the odds are stacked against cancer clone emergence by the interplay of chance and the restraints of DNA repair and cell death. The window of cancerous opportunity is really quite small.

Legacies of leaks?

The atomic bombs did much to acquaint the world with the hazards of ionizing radiation. But more than that, radiation became a very dirty word and a fear of its invisible tyranny was entrenched. Peaceful uses of atomic energy became suspect and doubts were not unreasonably fuelled by leaks, cover-ups, and suggestions of increases in childhood leukaemias and other cancers in the vicinity of installations. Irrespective of the commercial and environmental arguments for or against nuclear power, there is remarkably little persuasive evidence that, at least in recent times, the activities of nuclear fuel production or reprocessing plants increase local cancer rates. The monitored levels of radioactive release are below those that naturally exist in our environment. Leukaemia clusters do exist around one or two of such plants but there are other explanations. A colleague, Ray Cartwright, has a map which shows possible clusters of leukaemia based around sites in the UK labelled simply as 'military establishments'. The latter turn out to be derelict medieval forts and the apparent association is an illusion conjured up by chance. Other clusters, such as the one in the village of Seascale near the nuclear fuel reprocessing plant at Sellafield in the UK, are real but have been more plausibly explained by epidemiologist Leo Kinlen as reflecting unusual demographic features that have promoted childhood leukaemia via infection.[9] I'm not saying that nuclear plants can pose no danger in terms of cancer. Clearly the potential is there, but constrained, and one's confidence in the degree of constraint is contingent upon effective safety legislation, fail-safe devices, and monitoring.

There will also be a small but finite chance that a disaster will happen, aided and abetted by human error. Chernobyl is the obvious case in point. The explosion released large quantities of radioactive caesium and iodine into the air, plumes of which drifted downwind over much of the continent of Europe and Scandinavia. The impact in terms of cancer is not however what you might have anticipated from radiation folklore. There really is no evidence for any increases in childhood leukaemia in the most exposed areas despite popular press reports to the contrary. There is a significant increase in thyroid cancer in young individuals whose thyroid glands concentrated the inhaled radioactive iodine. No other excess cancers in children or adults have been reported, neither would they be expected from the nature and dose of radioactive substances released. Hard to believe I've been a paid-up member of Greenpeace isn't it?

But let's not let the Russians off the hook. At the time of writing, new stories are emerging from the old Soviet Union of regions in some of the southern republics where nuclear bomb test explosions may have left a devastating legacy of very high level environmental contamination and increased cancer rates. We'll doubtless hear more about this. But there have been other similar calamities perpetrated by the incompetence or negligence of the old Soviet industrial regime; Chernobyl was not the only nuclear power plant accident. An explosion in 1957 at the Mayak nuclear facility in Chelyabinsk in the Southern Urals resulted in radioactive contamination of the surrounding area, including the local Techa river – the same river that had served both as a deliberate dump for high-level radioactivity and a repository of leaks for several years before the accident. Several thousand occupants of villages along the river and in the flight path of the explosive release were resettled but may have taken with them a package of mutations and cancer risk. One analysis suggests that exposure of the population may have been as high as 4 Grays, and that this has significantly raised the subsequent incidence of leukaemia in the region, as would be anticipated from the consequences of the Japanese atomic bomb. It now appears that the Mayak complex has been the single most woeful planetary polluter with radioactivity; the surrounding river, lakes, and countryside receiving some five times more leakage than all 500 atmospheric nuclear tests, the Chernobyl accident, and Sellafield nuclear plant put together.

Addendum: animals as patients

'Are brute creatures subject to any disease resembling cancer in the human body? ... When this question is decided, we may enquire what class of animals is chiefly subject to cancer; the wild or the domesticated ... This investigation may lead to much philosophical amusement and useful information; particularly it may tell us how far the prevalence or frequency of cancer may depend upon the manners and habits of life.'

(Query number 10 (of 13) in the research agenda of the Society for Investigating the Nature and Cure of Cancer, Cancer Research Society, Edinburgh, 1806)

If it is correct that the potential for cancer is indigenous to the genetic blueprint of multicellular organisms and its high prevalence in *Homo sapiens* is an unfortunate by-product of our 'success' and exotic social structures and lifestyles, what then of cancer in other species?

Most animals, both vertebrate and invertebrate, have benign tumours and in some cases invasive cancers; even plants can have bacteria-induced tumours. These, we can safely assume, have existed long before *Homo sapiens* stood up and strode forth on the planet. Accurate estimates of incidence rates, especially in feral species, are not available although one might expect smaller, short-lived animals to have a relatively low risk. Cancer has been recorded in most species of captive mammals in zoos, but the incidence rates, even in ageing primates, appear very low in comparison with similar cancer types in humans.[10] It is then interesting to consider circumstances where cancer incidence in animals is high. Here are a few – all attributable to human interference or social engineering with the biology of another species:-

1 Genetically inbred and domesticated dogs have many types of cancer but especially breast cancer in bitches.

2 A high level of mammary and endometrial or uterine cancer in captive wild felids (tigers, lions, and so on) fed oral contraceptives (progestins).

3 'Socialized', domesticated, or artificially herded and inbred cattle, cats, and chickens all have virus-induced leukaemias. Bovine leukaemia is particularly interesting in this respect. This virus-induced cancer is endemic in cattle but is found at high rates in association with the activities of vets and husbandry methods, especially high-density over-winter housing. It turns out that in the past at least, vets have inadvertently recycled the

bovine virus involved here via re-use of syringes – a harbinger of human disasters with HIV.

4   Cattle put out to pasture on impoverished but bracken-rich soils – and oesophageal cancer.

5   Battery hens inundated with artificial light have very high rates of ovarian tumours.

6   Chickens that share the same diet as their Chinese keepers share a similar high rate of oesophageal (or for them, gullet) cancer. Fungal contamination and dietary insufficiencies may be part of the explanation.

7   Melanomas in horses bred to be white.

8   Epidemics of liver cancer in hatchery fish that had been fed with stored food contaminated with fungal aflatoxin.

9   Aquatic animals exposed to high levels of pollutants and mutagens; for example, molluscs in polluted estuaries have a significant incidence of tumours.

Welcome to our world.

CHAPTER 23

FINALE: CAUSE, COMPLEXITY, AND THE EVOLUTIONARY RUB

Both the biologist and the physical scientist need to reckon with historical legacies to explain any real-world phenomenon.

(George Williams, 1985)

The composite and probabilistic nature of risk for cancer, plus its extended time frame of evolutionary development, poses the major intellectual obstacle in understanding causation for the public and professionals alike. The ingredients and pattern of the composite are different for each type of cancer and, even for a single type of cancer, risk factors can vary in weight or importance. This is not intuitively easy to grasp given past false presumptions about disease causality. There is often a tacit assumption that not only can and should causation in cancer be formally and indisputably provable but that singular causes must exist and that these are both necessary and sufficient for the disease. This is simplistic and it is wrong.

Causation can be inferred as 'the most probable explanation' but it is extra-ordinarily difficult, if not impossible, to prove culpability beyond doubt. Moreover, since all cancers are multifactorial in origin and can arise via alternative causal mechanisms, the necessary and sufficient criterion is entirely inappropriate for cancer – as it is for the causation of most of our ailments. There just is not any all-encompassing and exclusive grip between particular causes and effects when it comes to cancer. Take the least ambiguous case: smoking is the major factor in lung cancer but it is not the only component in the causal pathway and clearly lung cancer can in special situations, develop via other insults and in the absence of cigarette tar. There is no singular cause of cancer, just as there is not, and is unlikely to be, a singular cure.

What we have in cancer is a plethora of causal pathways or networks within which risk is always a net product of positive and negative factors influencing the roulette wheel of cell proliferation, cell death, and mutation. Add together the diversity of disease, the multiplicity of risk factors, the time frames, plus the ubiquitous role of chance and it really is not at all surprising that epidemiological studies often struggle to arrive at consistent or unambiguous conclusions. We are fortunate indeed that so much can be reasonably inferred from such research. Chance and uncertainty pervade the cancer narrative and we are uncomfortable with this knowledge. As was said in the context of the BSE and other contemporary health scares, the trouble is we've replaced the certainty of religion with the uncertainty of science.

It is possible now however to distil this biological complexity into a general

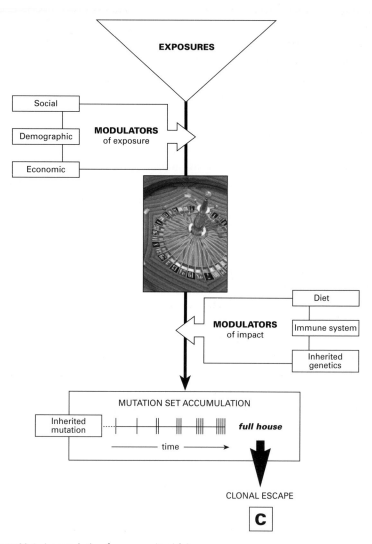

Figure 23.1 A prescription for composite risk in cancer.

picture of cancer causation in which our life-styles, environmental or 'internal' exposures, our variable genetics plus chance all interact to compound risk. This then provides us with a framework within which the peculiarities of individual cancers can be appreciated. Causation, for say breast cancer, seen in this light is still complex but not a mysterious, arcane, or impenetrable process. Figure 23.1 is an attempt to illustrate such a scheme. Exposures lead to increased mutations in DNA that can either initiate a cancerous clone or contribute to successive steps in its evolutionary progress. Tobacco carcinogens, for example, probably do both. The exposures can be external (for example, a virus) or endogenous (for example, hormones) but do not have direct access to DNA. They are subject to multiple modulators that operate either at the level of the exposure itself or downstream close to where the exposure impacts directly or indirectly on the integrity of DNA. Modulators include what are often referred to as 'lifestyle' factors, but these need to be considered in their historical and social context, not just as personal idiosyncrasies.

Particular patterns of exposures and modulators may operate as dominant but non-exclusive generators of cancer. All channel eventually into the same biological mechanism. The exposures involved and the 'targeted' tissue, cells, and genes differ, and cancer outputs vary, but in principle an equivalent network of risk factors and modulators operates in each case. The occasional product, a cancer clone, is itself assembled and selected to emerge over time by the same Darwinian ground rules as evolution itself. And the joker in the pack remains chance – the random ingredient that pervades cancer and evolution at every level.

When we posit, within this framework, the key question of why cancer is so common in human societies, albeit in different guises at different times and places, then the evolutionary and historical perspectives loom large. The proximal mechanics of cancer, mutation or genetic recombination and clonal cell selection, are intrinsic design features of biological systems that antedate human societies by more than a billion years. These attributes have been harnessed and exploited by evolutionary processes to provide the diversity and resilience upon which selective forces in changing environments operate to engineer both simple and complex bodies for survival and reproductive success. But the trade-off has to be an inherent risk of mutation empowering clonal emancipation and cancer. And as long as this only manifests itself as a chronic disorder endangering post-reproductive life, there is no negative selective pressure.

Many of the relevant exposures and negative modulators in cancer causation are the flip side of what were originally – for an emerging hominid species, subject over millennia to Darwinian fitness selection – advantageous attributes. These include selection for hormonally driven fertility, with persistently primed breasts, ovaries, uteruses, and prostates; some degree of promiscuity (in males at least); pale skins (for whatever reasons) in northerly folk; a propensity for periodic Bacchanalian bingeing and energy storage in fat; and longevity. And last but not least, an insatiably curious, risk-taking, tinkering, and entrepreneurial personality. These were all adaptations that engendered survival – reproductive and colonial ascendancy in particular ecological and social conditions. As always in evolution, the winning hand is dictated by the local circumstances that prevail at the time, with no eye for the future: context is everything.

But circumstances change. And, far more than any other species, we have manipulated and changed our habitats and behaviour. The social and environmental circumstances that spawned selective advantage have changed almost beyond recognition. Alternatively, down in the genes, remarkably little has stirred. For a start, the honourable *H. sapiens* has only been on the field around 10 000 generations, with just 400 generations since the pivotal agricultural and social changes in the Neolithic period some 10 000 years ago. Just a blinking of the evolutionary eye. And much of our current behavioural mores that we take for granted have only become entrenched or widespread over a few generations during the twentieth century.

For sure some selection via genetic variation has occurred over past millennia. This will have included adaptively neutral selection of individuals who were colonizers of new territories and therefore founders of subsequent generations. Natural selection will have operated *against* individuals who inherited fatal conditions that strike early in life, and *for* those whose immune systems were best equipped to restrain the ravages of plagues. The geneticist and polymath, J B S Haldane, was surely correct in suggesting that infections have been the most powerful 'natural' selective pressure acting on human populations. Other selective forces may have been at play manipulating the frequency of genetic variants. For example, those who could best detoxify naturally occurring plant carcinogens might accrue survival and therefore reproductive advantage. Natural selection could operate to indirectly reduce risk of cancer later in life *if*, say, the carcinogens involved were also toxic to the developing foetus. But, overall, these changes do little to alter our genetic adaptability in the face of altered and, in some cases, exotic lifestyles and exposures.

You might suppose that if our tissues and cells had been less efficiently programmed by evolution to frustrate cancerous proclivities and if cancer itself was a more acute, potent, and rapid assault on health, then the problem might have been resolved by Darwinian selection by now. But therein lies the rub: evolution has by and large taken care of this problem. The beneficial attributes of clonal expansion are thoroughly exploited and regulated for the ultimate benefit of reproductive success and the inbuilt trade-off or legacy is a set of chronic diseases that are only of real concern for a very idiosyncratic species that has changed the rules of the game.

Our cells and tissues have been set up over millions of years to be resilient in the face of insult – to expect it in fact. Still, over decades of chronic challenge, the inherent design limitations of the system come to the fore and a dominant clone may emerge from its ancient hide. And paradoxically, it is the very properties that endow our tissues with resilience and adaptability that generate, when subverted by mutation, clonal escapees able to wreck the body habitat; a cancerous 'catch 22'. And, fortunately or unfortunately, however you care to look at it, the cancerous catastrophes usually occur after we have served our prime biological (that is reproductive) function. But we are still hanging around, giving time for the improbable to happen. This deleterious and delayed penalty of our biology is now wholly invisible to natural selection. As far as nature is concerned, our cancers are, by and large, a non-issue.

It is obvious now that not only is there a network of causal factors 'causing' cancer but the essential features of the networks are historically and operationally multilayered. They have been assembled, piecemeal, over time spans ranging from decades to millions of years of evolutionary and social history as a deep and stratified legacy of what it takes to be a winner. Assembled, sustained, and periodically embellished with adaptive tricks in single-celled explorers; multicellular, corporate-bodied creatures; mammals; hominid primates; palaeolithic fire-making man; and, in more recent millennia, man the hairless one, the itinerant tinkerer and gambler. And now? Man the chimaera – the engineer, the fat pedant, and fabulous flyer; the genie that can clone his and her genes but remains subjugated to their vagaries.

The evolutionary perspective for cancer may be one of extraordinary antiquity and complexity but a similar theme runs through most of our diseases. Man has always inadvertently helped orchestrate the ecology of his diseases by his insatiable curiosity, migratory explorations, and dietary experiments. There is a sense in which all our ailments and particularly our 'modern' chronic disorders are reflections of design limitations, delayed trade-offs, and nature–nurture mismatches. They are part of the natural scheme of things even if we would like to believe that we have been sculptured to perfection. It is only quite recently that this evolutionary focus has been brought to bear on some of the major afflictions of modern societies – cardiovascular disease, diabetes, obesity, neurodegenerative conditions, and novel or re-emergent infectious diseases.

Randolph Nesse, a far-sighted physician, and George Williams, an eminent evolutionary biologist, have been prominent and eloquent proponents of this line and coined the term 'Evolutionary' or 'Darwinian Medicine' for this view of health and disease. Seen in this light, the predominant cancers of Western-ized societies (skin cancer, colon, prostate, breast, and lung carcinomas in particular) are part of a pattern of chronic, slow-acting degenerative conditions that emerge to pathological prominence mostly in post-reproductive life and whose current prevalence owes much to the discord between a 'modern' post-industrial lifestyle and a genetic prescription that tuned our biology and behaviour for conditions prevailing more than 10 000 years ago. In the vivid phraseology of anthropologist S Boyd Eaton, we are stone-agers in the fast lane.

And we've certainly been sprinting through the twentieth century. More-over, the whole social process and its malignant consequences has been reiterated as indigenous or native populations have been persuaded to mimic or adopt our 'modern' lifestyles. From this, some benefits have undoubtedly accrued but so too has a legacy of increasing lung, colo-rectal, and breast cancers in urbanized black Africans, Canadian Inuits, and others.

Despite the magnitude of this cancer toll, it is somewhat parochial and short-sighted to view it as a unique product of contemporary and affluent Western societies. Clearly we have been indulging in the behaviour versus biology conflict for many hundreds or a few thousand years in the form of dietary experiments, as the antiquity of oesophageal and stomach cancer testifies. Other cancers (those of viral or bacterial origin) reflect the perennial, oscil-lating conflict between ourselves and our microbes – outcomes influenced greatly by demographic changes in population structure and mobility. And only a minority of our current cancers are exclusive derivatives of twentieth-century technology.

In the main, the cancers that plague the Western or developed world today have been with us for centuries in one form or another. What modernity has provided is a rapid commercial and social expansion of risky attributes in a population otherwise enjoying longevity – an escalation of long-running mismatches. And, in the train of our startling progress, there are paradoxical penalty charges; a price to pay. But that price is not a fixed charge; there's a variable rate of cancer subtype incidence and outcome, related to scales of poverty and affluence. On the plus side, 90 per cent of the debt could, if we really set to it, be cancelled or deferred.

By now the reader will agree, I hope, that we have a highly plausible ex-planation for the causation of cancer. Not exactly the simple explanation that Susan Sontag anticipated, but a unitary explanation nonetheless. So no, it isn't your job, your stressful lifestyle, your genes, your diet, just bad luck, or an act of God that's to blame: a multilayered web of exposures and modifiers is involved. And, by and large, this network is a construct of very long-running evolutionary contests and problem solving, human history, and social engineering – heavily garnished in more recent centuries and decades with commercial and political imperatives, and pervaded throughout by chance.

Setting fire to it ... again

So how much credence do you give to the idea that so many factors can contribute to causal mechanisms and risk of cancer? Maybe it seems counter-intuitive, absurd, and contrary to real-life experiences or to what you see in the movies. But is it really so odd? Engineers and accident investigators are familiar with the chaotic and sometimes extravagant consequences that can follow from a collision of circumstances – historical design limitations, a stuck valve, human error, and pure chance. They are familiar with the non-linear and sometimes tortuous relationships between cause and effect in complex systems. So consider if you will, and as a parallel, the 'cause' of something non-medical that we are familiar with. An accidental fire is an apt metaphor.

Forest fires have been occurring sporadically ever since there were forests, and millions of years before we either planted or destroyed them. Fiery landscape scarring may even have a beneficial, regenerating effect on vegetation which some plants, the Eucalyptus species in particular, have become adept at exploiting. But the human talent for pyromechanics can modify the causal pathway and the risk. An effective agent for a forest fire might well be a carelessly dropped cigarette, though other agents of ignition, both man-made and natural, are obviously possible. The risk or impact imposed by the local source of heat will be influenced or modified by the type or species of vegetation on which it just by chance happened to fall, the season, whether or not it had rained recently, which way the wind (if any) was blowing, the presence or absence of non-inflammable barriers to dissemination (for example, a stream) and the possibility of early detection and intervention. By and large, the rare outcome – a raging fire – is then a chance conglomeration of sequential events, the most proximal components of which disguise the multiple and often remote historical contingencies involved.

You may find such multifaceted causal explanation tiresome, but it is undeniably a reasonable portrayal of the reality. And from this understanding, at least for accidental fires, obvious strategies to restrain their incidence or reduce their impact can emerge. Similarly, once one comprehends how the activities of cells and genes have been engineered by evolutionary selection, then the multiplicity of components contributing to risk and the probabilistic nature of outcome in cancer is exactly what one would expect.

These highly variable inputs do however include identifiable, major components and channel into common molecular and cellular events that drive the evolution of cancer by natural selection. There is therefore a unified and highly plausible mechanism at play. The challenge in unravelling the cancer process is then to embrace the complexity but give some weight to the major agents or modulators of risk in each main subtype of cancer and then to identify where, within the dynamic pathway of causation, intervention is likely to have a significant impact. Real-world practicalities – social acceptability, vested interests, political imperatives, and cost effectiveness then all come into play. I will discuss some of the options in the final section of this book but it's obvious that modifying some of our social habits and structures is likely to be more effective than tinkering with one's genes.

NOTES TO PART THREE

1 But not all agree. Some scientists subscribe to the 'Grandmother' selection idea. The gist of this is that during human evolution, grandmothers that provided succour and support to their children's children might facilitate the selection of genes that enhanced longevity.

2 Some anthropologists have recently proposed that the 'invention' of cooking plant tubers (yams and other potato-like subterranean starch-storage vessels) was a major turning point in hominid evolution some 1.8 million years ago, providing a rich source of calories and also spawning selection of important behavioural traits. But the idea may be 'half-baked' – see Pennici E (1999) *Science*, **283**:2004–5 for commentary. Others speculate that the control of fire had a significant impact on human evolution. Since it was an inherently dangerous or lethal activity it might, so argues Claire Russell, have provided selective pressure for bigger, smarter brains, and against coarse body hair (that is, for nakedness). Chimpanzees may have missed the boat in both fire making and linguistic skills, so Russell also intriguingly proposes, because of their laryngeal incapacity to blow out – see Russell C (1978) *Biol Hum Affairs*, **43**:14–20.

3 After reading this chapter, perhaps you can hazard a guess. A prize for the best answer.

4 There is at present no accurate way, or algorithm, to compute risk of breast cancer, or any other cancer for that matter; but guidelines are emerging. The National Cancer Institute has developed software, available on disk, called the 'Breast Cancer Risk Assessment Tool'. This is intended primarily for health care providers and suggests a way to calculate approximate risk of breast cancer developing over the following years. Parameters given weight include reproductive and family history, race, and age – but not diet or exercise use.

5 The underlying premise here is that all current *H. sapiens* did originate somewhere in East Africa some 150 000 to 250 000 years ago. Whilst this is the prevailing hypothesis, not everyone subscribes to this 'out of Africa' idea.

6 This idea was developed by W Farnsworth Loomis (see Loomis WF (1967) *Science*, **157**:501–6). For other ideas on the possible evolutionary signifi-

cance of skin colour see Diamond J (1991) *The rise and fall of the third chimpanzee*, Radius Publishing, UK; Jones S (1996) *In the blood*, Harper Collins, London; and Deol MS (1975) *Ann Hum Genet Lond*, **38**:501–3.

7 Reported by OB Urteaga and GT Pack in *Cancer* (1966), **19**:607–10. In their very brief description, the authors mention seven mummies but it is not clear from their ambiguous wording if all or several had melanoma. Remaining skin on the mummies was also said to have 'rounded melanotic masses' but unfortunately no photographs of these were provided. This material is no longer available for scrutiny and the diagnosis remains uncertain. There is also a possibility that the mummies studied were around a 1000 years old, not the 2400 years suggested in the original report (S Guillan, personal communication to author).

8 For a useful potted history of sooty chimneys, sweeps, and their warts in England, see Henry SA (1946) *Cancer of the scrotum in relation to cccupation*, Oxford University Press. Figure 21.1 is from this source. Two hundred years after Ramazzini's 'Diatribe', Thomas Oliver edited a similar but more voluminous and well-documented survey entitled *Dangerous trades* (1902), John Murray Publishers, London. In this report, chimney sweeps are recorded as having a higher rate of cancer than men employed in any other trade in England, a high level of lung diseases, and overall high mortality rate. In this respect it perhaps is not entirely surprising that they were also reported as being four times more likely (than the average tradesman) to indulge 'intemperance' and twice as likely to commit suicide.

9 Apparent clusters of cancers in children, have a particular potency in generating alarm. One of the best established cases is an old one – a cluster of eight cases of leukaemia in children living in the same parish of the Niles suburb of Chicago in 1957–60. The cause was never established but is most likely to have involved an infectious episode. In other situations, such as the Woburn (Massachussetts) case (spawning the book and movie 'A Civil Action'), environmental chemical contamination has been indicted by action groups but unproven. The most recent leukaemia cluster (in adults this time) involves three professors and one former student of the Mozarteum Music School in Salzburg – a statistical fluke, contaminated air conditioning, Saltière's revenge? Who knows? It is extraordinarily difficult to prove causality in isolated, one-off incidences such as these.

10 I am grateful to Dr Dick Montali of the National Zoological Park, Washington DC and Professor David Onions of Glasgow University for directing me to useful sources of information on cancer in feral, captive, and domesticated animals. Some useful references include Jubb KVF, Kennedy PC, Palmer N, eds. (1993) *Pathology of domestic animals*. Vol. 3,

4th edn. Academic Press, San Diego; Montali RJ and Migaki G, eds. (1980) *Pathology of zoo animals.* Smithsonian Institution Press, Washington DC; National Cancer Institute (July 1969) *Neoplasms and related disorders of invertebrate and lower vertebrate animals.* Monograph 31. US Department of Health, Education, and Welfare, Public Health Service, National Cancer Institutes, Bethesda; Harrenstien LA, Munson L, Seal US, American Zoo and Aquarium Association Mammary Cancer Study Group (1996) Mammary cancer in captive wide felids and risk factors for its development: a retrospective study of the clinical behaviour of 31 cases. *J Zoo Wildlife Med*, **27**:468–76.

FURTHER READING

General: cancer epidemiology, causal pathways, and aetiology

Adami H-O and Trichopoulos D, eds. (1998) *Progress in Enigmas in Cancer Epidemiology*, Seminars in cancer biology. Vol. 8, No. 4.

Doll R and Peto R (1981) *The causes of cancer.* Oxford University Press, Oxford.

(1996) Harvard report on cancer prevention. Vol. 1: causes of human cancer. *Cancer Causes and Control*, **7(suppl)**.

International Agency for Research on Cancer (IARC) *Monographs on the evaluation of carcinogenic risks to humans.* IARC, Lyon. (A large series of careful and authoritative analyses and risk assessments of various biological, chemical, and physical agents that may be involved in cancer causation.)

Lewontin RC (1993) *The doctrine of DNA biology as ideology.* Penguin Books.

Liechtenstein P, Holm NV, Verkasalo PK, Iliadou A, Kaprio J, Koskenvuo M, *et al.* (2000) Environmental and heritable factors in the causation of cancer. *N Engl J Med*, **343**:78–85.

Parkin DM, Pisani P, Ferlay J (1999) Estimates of the worldwide incidence of 25 major cancers in 1990. *Int J Cancer*, **80**:827–41.

Perera FP (1996) Uncovering new clues to cancer risk. *Scientific American*, **May**:54–62.

Root-Bernstein (1993) Evolution and emergent properties. In: *New frontiers in cancer causation* (Iverson OH, ed.), pp. 1–14. Taylor and Francis Publishers, Washington DC.

Schottenfeld D and Fraumeni JF, eds. (1996) *Cancer epidemiology and prevention.* 2nd edn. Oxford University Press, New York.

Taubes G (1995) Epidemiology faces its limits. *Science*, **269**:164–9.

Tomatis L (1995) Socioeconomic factors and human cancer. *Int J Cancer*, **62**:121–5.

Trichopoulos D, Petridou E, Lipworth L, Adami H-O (1997) In: *Cancer: principles and practice of oncology* (DeVita VT, Hellman S, Rosenberg SA). 5th edn, pp. 231–51. Lippincott-Raven Publishing, Philadelphia.

Ageing and cancer

Cohen HJ (1994) Biology of aging as related to cancer. *Cancer*, **74**:2092–210.

Balducci L, Lyman GH, Ershler WB, eds. (1998) *Comprehensive geriatric oncology*. Harwood Academic.

Pennisi E (1996) Premature aging gene discovered. *Science*, **272**:193–4.

Peto R, Roe FJC, Lee PN, Levy L, Clack J (1975) Cancer and ageing in mice and men. *Br J Cancer*, **32**:411–26.

Simpson AJG and Camargo AA (1998) Evolution and the inevitability of human cancer. *Sem Cancer Biol*, **8**:439–46.

Tollefsbol TO and Cohen HJ (1984) Werner's syndrome: an underdiagnosed disorder resembling premature aging. *Age*, **7**:75–88.

Fire making

Brink AS (1957) The spontaneous fire-controlling reactions of two chimpanzee smoking addicts. *South African J Science*, **April**:241–7.

Frazer JG (1930) *Myths of the origin of fire*. Macmillan, London.

Goudsblom J (1993) *Fire and civilization*. Allen Lane, Penguin Press, London.

James SR (1989) Hominid use of fire in the lower and middle pleistocene. *Curr Anthropology*, **30**:1–26.

Perlès C (1977) *Préhistoire du feu*. Masson, Paris.

Tobacco and lung cancer

BR Med J (whole issue on 'Towards a smoke free world'), 5 August 2000, No. 7257.

Count Corti (1931) *A history of smoking*. (Translated by Paul England). G G Harrap Publishers, Bombay and Sydney. (A remarkably erudite, informative, and entertaining book. Some of the historical tales recounted in 'And then you set fire to it?' derive from this source.)

Denissenko MF, Pao A, Tang M, Pfeifer GP (1996) Preferential formation of benzo[a]pyrene adducts at lung cancer mutational hotspots in *P53*. *Science*, **274**:430–2.

Doll R and Hill AB (1950) Smoking and carcinoma of the lung. Preliminary report. *BMJ*, **2**:739–48.

Doll R, Peto R, Wheatley K, Gray R, Sutherland I (1994) Mortality in relation to smoking: 40 years' observations on male British doctors. *BMJ*, **309**:901–9.

Erichsen-Brown C (1979) Medicinal and other uses of North American plants. A historical survey with special reference to the Eastern Indian Tribes. General Publishing Co., Toronto.

Gao Y-T, Blot WJ, Zheng W, Ershow AG, Hsu CW, Levin LI, *et al.* (1987) Lung cancer among Chinese women. *Int J Cancer*, **40**:604–9.

Hecht SS (1999) Tobacco smoke carcinogens and lung cancer. *J Natl Cancer Inst*, **91**:1194–210.

Hoffman FL (1931) Cancer and smoking habits. *Ann Surg*, **93**:50–67.

James I (republished 1954) *A counter-blaste to tobacco*. The Rodale Press, London. (A wonderfully scripted diatribe.)

Johnson DH, ed. (1977) Lung cancer. *Seminars in Oncology*, **vol. 24(4)**.

Mackay J (1996) Tobacco: the third world war. Advice from General Sun Tzu. *J Royal Coll Physicians*, **30**:360–5.

Peto R, Chen Z-M, Boreham J (1999) Tobacco—the growing epidemic. *Nature Med*, **5**:15–17.

Proctor RN (1996) The anti-tobacco campaign of the Nazis: a little known aspect of public health in Germany, 1933–45. *BMJ*, **313**:1450–3.

Redmond DG (1970) Tobacco and cancer: the first clinical report, 1761. *N Engl J Med*, **282**: 18–23.

Wynder EL and Graham EA (1950) Tobacco smoking as a possible etiologic factor in bronchogenic carcinoma. *J Am Med Assoc*, **143**:329–36.

Informative exposés of the tobacco industry and cancer

Glantz S, Slade J, Bero LA, Hanauer P, Barnes DE (1996) *The cigarette papers*. California Press, Berkeley.

Hilts PJ (1996) *Smokescreen. The truth behind the tobacco industry cover-up*. Addison-Wesley, Reading, MA.

Kluger R (1996) *Ashes to ashes. America's hundred-year cigarette war, the public health, and the unabashed triumph of Philip Morris*. Knopf, New York.

Breast cancer

Colditz GA and Frazier AL (1995) Models of breast cancer show that risk is set by events of early life: prevention efforts must shift focus. *Cancer Epidemiol, Biomarkers and Prevention*, **4**:567–71.

Couch FJ and Hartmann LC (1998) *BRCA1* testing – advances and retreats. *J Am Med Assoc*, **279**:955–6.

DeMoulin D (1983) *A short history of breast cancer*. Kluwer Publishers, Dordrecht, The Netherlands. (An excellent review of historical ideas on breast cancer.)

Eaton SB, Pike MC, Short RV, *et al.* (1994) Women's reproductive cancers in evolutionary context. *Quarterly Rev Biol*, **69**:353–67. (A series of reviews detailing some of the evolutionary ideas on breast cancer risk propounded by S Boyd Eaton and Malcolm Pike in particular.)

Galdikas BMF and Wood JW (1990) Birth spacing patterns in humans and apes. *Am J Physical Anthropol*, **83**:185–91.

Graham CE, ed. (1981) *Reproductive biology of the great apes*. Academic Press, New York.

Hankinson SE, Willett WC, Colditz GA, Hunter DJ, Michaud DS, Deroo B, *et al.* (1998) Circulating concentrations of insulin-like growth factor-I and risk of breast cancer. *Lancet*, **351**: 1393–6.

Henderson BE, Ross RK, Pike MC, Casagrande JT (1982) Endogenous hormones as a major factor in human cancer. *Cancer Res*, **42**:3232–9.

Hulka BS and Stark AT (1995) Breast cancer: cause and prevention. *Lancet*, **346**:883–7.

Jordan VC (1998) Designer estrogens. *Scientific American*, **October**: 36–43.

Kagawa Y (1978) Impact of Westernization on the nutrition of Japanese: changes in physique, cancer, longevity and centenarians. *Preventive Med*, **7**:205–17.

Kelsey JL, ed. (1993). Breast cancer. *Epidemiol Rev*, **vol. 15 (no. 1)**.

Konner M and Worthman C (1980) Nursing frequency, gonadal function, and birth spacing among !Kung hunter-gatherers. *Science*, **207**:788–91.

Land CE (1995) Studies of cancer and radiation dose among atomic bomb survivors. The example of breast cancer. *J Am Med Assoc*, **274**:402–7.

Light A and Saraf I (1997) *Rachel's daughers*. Light/Saraf Films (home video version), distributed by Women Make Movies, New York, USA.

Lipworth L (1995) Epidemiology of breast cancer. *Eur J Cancer Prevention*, **4**:7–30.

MacMahon B, Cole P, Brown J (1973) Etiology of breast cancer: a review. *J Natl Cancer Inst*, **50**:21–42.

Mezzetti M, La Vecchia C, Decarli A, Boyle P, Talamini R, Franceschi S (1998) Population attributable risk for breast cancer: diet, nutrition, and physical exercise. *J Natl Cancer Inst*, **90**:389–94.

Mustacchi P (1961) Ramazzini and Rigoni-Stern on parity and breast cancer. *Arch Int Med*, **108**:639–42.

Pike MC, Krailo MD, Henderson BE, Casagrande JT, Hoel DG (1983) 'Hormonal' risk factors, 'breast tissue age' and the age-incidence of breast cancer. *Nature*, **303**:767–70.

Risch HA, Weiss NS, Lyon JL, Daling JR, Liff JM (1983) Events of reproductive life and the incidence of epithelial ovarian cancer. *Am J Epidemiol*, **117**:128–39.

Shattuck-Eidens D, Oliphant A, McClure M, McBride C, Gupte J, *et al.* (1997) *BRCA1* sequence analysis in women at high risk for susceptibility mutations. *J Am Med Assoc*, **278**:1242–50.

Spencer Feigelson H, McKean-Cowdin R, Coetzee GA, Stram DO, Kolonel LN, Henderson BE (2001) Building a multigenetic model of breast cancer susceptibility: *CYP17* and *HSD17B1* are two important candidates. *Cancer Res*, **61**:785–9.

Stuart-Macadam P and Dettwyler KA (1996) *Breast feeding. Biocultural perspectives.* A de Gruyter Publishers, New York.

Symmers WStC (1968) Carcinoma of breast in trans-sexual individuals after surgical and hormonal interference with the primary and secondary sex characteristics. *BMJ*, **2**:83–5.

Szabo CI and King M-C (1997) Population genetics of *BRCA1* and *BRCA2*. *Am J Hum Genet*, **60**:1013–20.

Tokunaga M, Land CE, Tokuoka S, Nishimori I, Soda M, Akiba S (1994) Incidence of female breast cancer among atomic bomb survivors, 1950–1985. *Radiation Res*, **138**:209–23.

Yalom M (1997) *A history of the breast.* Alfred A Knopf, New York.

Prostate cancer

Bruce AW and Trachtenberg J, eds. (1987) *Adenocarcinoma of the prostate.* Springer-Verlag, London.

Cohen P (1998) Serum insulin-like growth factor-I levels and prostate cancer risk—interpreting the evidence. *J Natl Cancer Inst*, **90**:876–9.

Das S and Crawford ED, eds. (1993) *Cancer of the prostate.* Marcel Dekker Inc, New York.

Hebert JR, Hurley TG, Olendzki BC, Teas J, Ma Y, Hampl JS (1998)

Nutritional and socioeconomic factors in relation to prostate cancer mortality: a cross-national study. *J Natl Cancer Inst*, **90**:1637–47.

Karp JE, Chiarodo A, Brawley O, Kelloff GJ (1996) Prostate cancer prevention: investigational approaches and opportunities. *Cancer Res*, **56**:5547–56.

Makridakis NM, Ross RK, Pike MC, Crocitto LE, Kolonel LN, Pearce CL, *et al.* (1999) Association of mis-sense substitution in *SRD5A2* gene with prostate cancer in African–American and Hispanic men in Los Angeles, USA. *Lancet*, **354**:975–8.

Ross RK, Pike MC, Coetzee GA, Reichardt JKV, Yu MC, Feigelson H, *et al.* (1998) Androgen metabolism and prostate cancer: establishing a model of genetic susceptibility. *Cancer Res*, **58**,4497–504.

Sakr WA, Haas GP, Cassin BF, Pontes JE, Crissman JD (1993) The frequency of carcinoma and intraepithelial neoplasia of the prostate in young male patients. *J Urology*, **150**:379–85.

Sidney S, Quesenberry CP, Friedman GD, Tekawa IS (1997) Marijuana use and cancer incidence (California, United States). *Cancer Causes and Control*, **8**:722–8.

Steele R, Lees REM, Kraus AS, Rao C (1971) Sexual factors in the epidemiology of cancer of the prostate. *J Chron Dis*, **24**:29–37.

Cervical cancer and human papilloma viruses

Bauer HM, Ting Y, Greer CE, Chambers JC, Tashiro CJ, Chimera J, Reingold A, *et al.* (1991) Genital human papillomavirus infection in female university students as determined by a PCR-based method. *J Am Med Assoc*, **265**:472–7.

Brinton LA, Reeves WC, Brenes MM, Herrero R, Gaitan E, Tenorio F, *et al.* (1989) The male factor in the etiology of cervical cancer among sexually monogamous women. *Int J Cancer*, **44**: 199–203.

Cuzick J, Terry G, Ho L, Hollingworth T, Anderson M (1992) Human papillomavirus type 16 DNA in cervical smears as predictor of high-grade cervical cancer. *Lancet*, **339**:959–60.

Ellis JRM, Keating PJ, Baird J, Hounsell EF, Renouf DV, Rowe M, *et al.* (1995) The association of an HPV16 oncogene variant with HLA-B7 has implications for vaccine design in cervical cancer. *Nature Med*, **1**:464–9.

Franco EL (1995) Cancer causes revisited: human papillomavirus and cervical neoplasia. *J Natl Cancer Inst*, **87**:779–80.

Morris JDH, Eddleston ALWF, Crook T (1995) Viral infection and cancer. *Lancet*, **346**:754–8.

Shingleton HM and Orr JW, eds. (1995) *Cancer of the cervix*. JB Lippincott Co, Philadelphia.

Thomas DB, Ray RM, Pardthaisong T, Chutivongse S, Koetsawang S, Silpisornkosol S, *et al.* (1996) Prostitution, condom use, and invasive squamous cell cervical cancer in Thailand. *Am J Epidemiol*, **143**:779–86.

Other infectious microbes and cancer

Gross L, ed. (1983) *Oncogenic viruses.* 3rd edn. Pergamon Press, New York.

Parsonnet J, Ed (1999) Microbes and Malignancy. Oxford University Press, New York.

Newton R, Beral V, Weiss RA, eds. (1999) *Infections and human cancer.* Cold Spring Harbor Laboratory Press, Cold Spring Harbor.

Scheiman JM and Cutler AF (1999) *Helicobacter pylori* and gastric cancer. *Am J Med*, **106**: 222–6.

Sun, skin colour, and cancer

Ariel IM, ed. (1981) *Malignant melanoma.* Appleton-Century-Crofts, New York.

Armstrong BK and Kricker A (1994) Cutaneous melanoma. In: *Cancer surveys, volume 19: trends in cancer incidence and mortality*, pp. 219–40. Imperial Cancer Research Fund, London.

Elwood JM (1996) Melanoma and sun exposure. *Sem Oncol*, **23**:650–66.

Harris CC (1996) Molecular epidemiology of basal cell carcinoma. *J Natl Cancer Inst*, **88**: 315–17.

Leffell DJ and Brash DE (1996) Sunlight and skin cancer. *Scientific American*, **July**:38–43.

Pennisi E (1996) Gene linked to commonest cancer. *Science*, **272**:1583–4.

Yarbro JW, Bornstein RS, Mastrangelo MJ, eds. (1996) Melanoma. *Seminars in Oncology*, **Vol. 23**, No. 6.

Diet and cancer risk

Block G (1992) The data support a role for antioxidants in reducing cancer risk. *Nutrition Rev*, **50**: 207–13.

Blot WJ, Li J-Y, Taylor PR, Guo W, Dawsey S, Wang G-Q, *et al.* (1993) Nutrition intervention trials in Linxian, China: supplementation with specific vitamin/mineral combinations, cancer incidence, and disease-specific mortality in the general population. *J Natl Cancer Inst*, **85**: 1483–92.

Cheng KK, Day NE, Duffy SW, Lam TH, Fok M, Wong J (1992) Pickled vegetables in the aetiology of oesophageal cancer in Hong Kong Chinese. *Lancet*, **339**:1314–18.

Correa P (1992) Human gastric carcinogenesis: a multistep and multifactorial process – first American Cancer Society Award lecture on cancer epidemiology and prevention. *Cancer Res*, **52**: 6735–40.

Eaton SB, Eaton III SB, Konner MJ (1997) Paleolithic nutrition revisited: a twelve-year retrospective on its nature and implications. *Eur J Clin Nutrition*, **51**:207–16.

Eaton SB, Konner M, Shostak M (1988) Stone agers in the fast lane: chronic degenerative diseases in evolutionary perspective. *Am J Med*, **84**:739–49.

Food, nutrition and the prevention of cancer: a global perspective (1997). World Cancer Research Fund in association with the American Institute for Cancer Research.

Frankel S, Gunnell DJ, Peters TJ, Maynard M, Davey Smith G (1998) Childhood energy intake and adult mortality from cancer: the Boyd Orr cohort study. *BMJ*, **316**:499–504.

Kaplan HS and Tsuchitani PJ (1978) *Cancer in China*. Alan R Liss Publishers, New York.

Milton K (1993) Diet and primate evolution. *Scientific American*, **August**, 70–7.

Muñoz N and Day NE (1996) Esophageal cancer. In: *Cancer epidemiology and prevention*. 2nd edn., pp. 681–706. Oxford University Press, New York.

O'Dea K (1991) Traditional diet and food preferences of Australian Aboriginal hunter-gatherers. *Phil Trans R Soc Lond B*, **334**:233–41.

Potter JD (1992) Reconciling the epidemiology, physiology, and molecular biology of colon cancer. *J Am Med Assoc*, **268**:1573–7.

Potter JD, Slattery ML, Bostick RM, Gapstur SM (1993) Colon cancer: a review of the epidemiology. *Epidemiologic Rev*, **15**:499–545.

Cancer risk from occupational, medicinal, and environmental exposures

Band P, ed. (1990) *Occupational cancer epidemiology*. Springer-Verlag, Berlin.

Bhatia S, Robison LL, Oberlin O, Greenberg M, Bunin G, Fossati-Bellani F, *et al.* (1996) Breast cancer and other second neoplasms after childhood Hodgkin's disease. *N Engl J Med*, **334**: 745–51.

Boice JD and Travis LB (1995) Body wars: effect of friendly fire (cancer therapy). *J Natl Cancer Inst*, **87**:705–6.

Butlin HT (1892) Three lectures on cancer of the scrotum in chimney-sweeps and others. *BMJ*, **2 July**:1–6.

Caufield C (1989) *Multiple exposures*. Secker & Warburg, London.

Doll R (1995) Hazards of ionising radiation: 100 years of observations on man. *Br J Cancer*, **72**:1339–49.

Enderle GJ and Friedrich K (1995) East German uranium miners (Wismut) – exposure conditions and health consequences. *Stem Cells*, **13(suppl 1)**:78–89.

Kossenko MM, Degteva MO, Vyushkova OV, Preston DL, Mabuchi K, Kozheurov VP (1997) Issues in the comparison of risk estimates for the population in the Techa river region and atomic bomb survivors. *Radiation Res*, **148**:54–63. For editorial commentaries on this environmental disaster, see Marshall E (1997), *Science*, **275**:1062 and Edwards SR (December 1997), *New Scientist*, p. 15.

Leitch A (1924) Mule-spinners' cancer and mineral oils. *BMJ*, **22 Nov**:941–4.

London NJ, Farmery SM, Will EJ, Davison AM, Lodge JPA (1995) Risk of neo-plasia in renal transplant patients. *Lancet*, **346**:403–6.

Pearce N, Matos E, Vanio H, Boffetta P, Kogevinas M, eds. (1994) *Occupational cancer in developing countries*. IARC Scientific Publications, No 129, Lyon.

Peto J, Hodgson JT, Matthews FE, Jones JR (1995) Continuing increase in mesothelioma mortality in Britain. *Lancet*, **345**:535–9.

Potts P (1775) Chirurgical observations relative to the cataract, the polypus of the nose, the cancer of the scrotum, the different kinds of ruptures, and the mortification of the toes and feet. *Tracts 92*. London. Hawes L, Clarke W, Collins R.

Ramazzini B (1964) *Diseases of workers*. Hafner Publishing Co., New York.

Schull WJ, ed. (1995) *Effects of atomic radiation*. Wiley-Liss, New York.

Southam AH and Wilson SR (1922) Cancer of the scrotum. *BMJ*, **18 Nov**:971–3.

PART FOUR

FINESSING THE CLONE

Cancer cannot be cured and will never be cured; but the world wants
to be fooled.

(Gui Patin, Dean of the Paris Medical Faculty, 1665)

Indeed a great deal of industrious work is being done (on cancer) …
but someone should have another bright idea.

(R Virchow, 1896)

I conclude, as I did seven years ago, that our decades of war against
cancer have been a qualified failure. Thank you.

(J C Bailar II at the Vice President's Cancer Panel Meeting, 1993)

I conclude that we are, for the most part, winning the fight against
cancer.

(Sir Richard Doll, 1990)

CHAPTER 24

TREATMENT: THE BLINDFOLDED MARKSMAN

The long history of cancer in human society is replete with exotic or bizarre treatments, quackery, and gallant failure. Radical intervention by the surgeon's knife has for centuries vied with the herbalist's less harrowing, if ineffective, remedies and when all else fails, there has been no shortage of the surreal:

> An example of a woman who had cancer of the breast, which was already so severe that eight holes had been eaten into it, and who recovered through the following expedient: She took eight frogs applied to the breast in a muslin bag, which attached themselves instantly thereto as firmly as leeches. When they had sucked to repletion, they dropped off in violent convulsions without the sucking causing pain. This was repeated until 20 frogs were used, which all from time to time, sucked until they died. And the breast was not only cured, but returned again to its normal size absolutely.
>
> *(From Kook-Koeck en Recepte Boek by E J Dijkman, Cape Colony, 1905)*

The more recent history of cancer treatment during the twentieth century has its share of quixotic sagas from miracle cures to outright fraud; a testament to both the entrepreneurial spirit and credulity of human beings. And it is no accident that this has been more pronounced in the USA than elsewhere. Millions of dollars have been spent by vulnerable and often desperate cancer patients beguiled by outrageous and bogus claims for efficacy or, at best, unsubstantiated anecdotes. The American constitution protects the right of individuals to exercise freedom of choice and similarly protects the right of news media to place their own slant on cancer stories. The US Food and Drugs Administration's (FDA) legal requirement for proven efficacy dangles the threat of prosecution over purveyors of useless or dangerous remedies – but there's always been a back door or failing that, another country. Infamous examples include Dr William F Koch's cancer treatment in the 1940s and 50s:

pure distilled water at 300 dollars an injection. Koch escaped condemnation at trial and retired to live in Brazil. A more bizarre but equally scandalous hoax was perpetrated in the 1950s by one, Henry Hoxsey. The secret formula for his herbal tonic as revealed in his book *You don't have to die* was discovered in 1840 by his great grandfather whose horse recovered from cancer of the leg after grazing in a field of mixed weeds. Hence the cocktail – prickly ash bark, red clover blossoms, barberry root, liquorice root, pokeweed, alfalfa, buckthorn bark, and burdock root – all dissolved in a common laxative. Delicious. The FDA finally stopped the activities of the Hoxsey clinic in the USA, but not until cancer patients had forked out an estimated 50 million dollars. Other notorious cases include, in the 1960s, Krebiozen's mineral oil and laetrile (a cyanide-containing extract of apricot kernels).

One of the ironies of these and many other cases was that the purveyors of ineffective remedies were often sustained by the staunch advocacy of patients themselves. These historical cases find a recent echo in Italy where Luigi Di Bella's cancer-curing cocktail has had politicians, the media, doctors, and patients in a frenzy. There has been a huge public demand for it, propelled by an anecdotal cure score that runs into thousands, so say the believers. Millions of dollars have been spent on clinical trials, now abandoned, but no credible evidence for efficacy has emerged. Di Bella is, allegedly, planning to sue his critics.

Not all such claims for curative cocktails are necessarily fraudulent, neither are they all detrimental or useless in terms of quality of life impact. What they signal is that an exploitable market for alternative remedies will persist as long as conventional medicine is perceived to be failing. But is it? We've certainly come to expect much more of our medical establishment and a great deal has been achieved. But the signals have been mixed and confusing: gallant failure in one ear and breakthrough hyperbole in the other. What is going on and does an evolutionary view of cancer have anything useful to contribute to the debate?

The high prevalence of cancer in our society is not for want of sustained and sometimes heroic attempts to eradicate it, by oncologists – and their patients. In the USA, billions of dollars have been expended since the 1970s in an attempt to beat cancer. This effort was set up and Presidentially inspired with much optimism and rhetoric. Comparisons were drawn with the Manhattan atomic bomb project, putting man on the moon, and, even, a 'medical Vietnam'. Unfortunately the underlying premises and state of knowledge at the time were sadly deficient, raised unrealistic hopes, and led inevitably to disappointment and scepticism. The quote above by Bailar, now at McGill University, reflected a common though not universally held view that very little had been achieved for 15 years of effort and huge sums of money. And

Americans don't take this sort of news lying down. But what are the facts? Has there been no improvement in treatment and cure rates?

In part, the confusion arises because of the way clinical results are presented. Mortality figures aren't quite the simple and unambiguous end point you might suppose. The prospects for death versus survival for a cancer will depend of course on the efficacy of treatment received but overall, the proportion surviving and the number of years of survival after a diagnosis will be influenced by diagnostic variables including cancer screening programmes that detect incipient cancers. Total death toll will also be modulated up or down, irrespective of treatment, by any alterations in real incidence levels (disallowing diagnostic variables). These factors can then distort appreciation of treatment success or failure. The bottom line is that the real incidence rate of several malignant cancers is up, others down; incidence figures are inflated by screening programmes but early intervention can improve prospects for survival. Finally, treatment success for more advanced or metastatic cancers has only been unequivocal in selected, and possibly biologically special, cases.

It is true that, as Bailar had insisted, progress in reducing overall mortality has up to now been slight but as Sir Richard Doll has persuasively argued, the overall statistics are misleading and not only because of the complications referred to above. Doll's analysis reveals that when individual cancer types are scrutinized, particularly for the younger age groups – which is where we might expect to see some benefit emerging first – then a more encouraging picture emerges. For some 14 types of cancer, there was a 10 per cent or more fall in mortality (in either males or females aged 20–44 years) in 1986–87 as compared with 1951–54 (in Europe and the USA). At the turn of the century, statistics from the UK suggest that chemotherapy, including tamoxifen, has had a significant beneficial impact on survival rates for breast cancer.

Hidden behind these mildly encouraging averages are some causes for concern. Success rates in controlling or eradicating major cancers vary significantly between and within Westernized countries. Why do women diagnosed with breast cancer in Scotland fare worse clinically than those in Cologne or Chicago? Why do native Americans in the USA come bottom of the 'ethnic' league table for cancer survival? There are a number of possible explanations but it seems that the screening, referral, diagnosis, and treatment practices do vary in availability and efficiency. Further improvements in cancer treatment could and should come from better organization with more emphasis on specialist centres. Access to optimal health care in cancer, as with other serious illnesses, ought not to be a geographical or social lottery in which the poorer, less educated sections of the community are the predominant losers.[1]

Other cancers show no beneficial change and some show actual increases in both incidence rates and mortality in the same younger age group. The latter includes cancers of the pancreas, oesophagus, bladder, and melanoma skin cancer. There are paradoxes here also. In the USA, more people are dying of melanoma than ever before but there have been real improvements in early diagnosis and eradication by surgery. In the 1950s, only 50 per cent of those with early-stage melanoma survived; today it's over 90 per cent. The explanation? Melanoma is five times more common now than it was 50 years ago; we haven't been able to keep pace with this increase.

The reasons for the diminished mortality in some cancers are also very mixed. Only part of the success is attributable to treatment with more effective chemotherapy – for choriocarcinoma, testicular cancer, childhood leukaemia, Hodgkin's disease, and paediatric kidney cancers in particular. And in these instances, success may have been possible for special and somewhat serendipitous biological reasons that I'll return to shortly. For the marked reduction in lung cancer in young males and for stomach cancer in Europe and the USA, the explanation and credit lies outside the clinic – fewer individuals are developing these cancers than previously.

Reductions in cigarette smoking amongst males are clearly responsible for the marked decline in lung cancer incidence. Changes in food preparation and preservation, combined perhaps with other dietary improvements are, at least in part, responsible for the reduced incidence of stomach cancer and perhaps for colo-rectal cancer also. Changing patterns of hygiene and infection in infancy may, as we have seen, also play a part in the decline of stomach cancer. The mortality from cervical carcinoma in the USA and western Europe has declined by some 50 per cent since 1960, but the incidence has actually increased during that period. The answer to this paradox is illuminating and sets an important precedent. We are no better at treating disseminated, malignant, cervical cancer now than before, but by introducing community-wide screening tests (the PAP smear) it is possible to 'catch' cancer clones on route to malignant independence and to dispose of them before they become intransigent invaders.

This analysis suggests a more balanced appraisal of our progress especially when placed alongside other very considerable advances in, for example, earlier diagnosis, tumour imaging, focused (conformal) radiotherapy, reconstructive surgery, supportive care, palliative treatment (including pain control), and counselling. There is much more to patient treatment, care, and management than attempting to clobber the clone. A diagnosis of cancer remains very unwelcome news but, in affluent countries at least, not as bad as at any time in the past. But, realistically, our progress in disease control and eradication has been at best modest for the major adult cancers and the statistics, however they are distilled, provide cold comfort for individual patients. By any measure, we still have a long way to go.

Escaping the axe: the trouble with natural selection

Let's take a closer, biological look at why cancer cells appear to out-manoeuvre the oncologists' heavy weaponry and escape through this critical bottleneck. It's a salutary lesson pervaded by the cold current of Darwinian logic.

Cancer is treated by surgery, radiation, and chemotherapy or, in the language of the cynic, by cutting, burning, and poisoning. It is a crude business. If tumours are relatively small, detectable, and in convenient sites, then surgeons can remove them, much as Leonides of Alexandria performed mastectomies for breast cancer some time ago (AD 180). That excision alone can eradicate the problem in some cases is not in doubt. But clearly it can and does fail. And it does so for what we can now see as an obvious problem: the fact that the tumour looks, both to the surgeon with knife poised and to the histopathologist peering down the microscope, to have discrete physical boundaries, provides illusory reassurance. Individual cancer cells can spread undetected beyond these confines to local and more distant territories. As they begin this voyage, they are invisible to traditional observational methods and may also elude detection by sophisticated whole-body scanning. The latter has a fine resolution down to a few cubic millimetres or so, but this requires one emigrant cell to have generated a million or more descendants in one spot in order for it to be visualized. Itinerant cancer cells wandering by themselves or generating modest numbers of descendants can only be unearthed by newer molecular techniques that exploit the cancer cells' mutations as identity tags. These more penetrating tools for digging in tissue or screening biological fluids (sputum, blood, urine) or faeces have yet to be utilized in the clinic. The real problem in cancer treatment comes from the spread of disease throughout and between tissues, which so often is covert and asymptomatic and therefore occurs before the problem can be recognized by patient or physician.

Once a cancer clone has evolved to this stage of territorial exploration, the knife is redundant and the blunter instruments of ionizing radiotherapy and chemotherapy with drug combinations have to be co-opted into action. These treatment modalities operate on the principle that any cell that has a very active metabolism and is rapidly dividing will be killed. You don't need a doctorate in biology to appreciate that this approach lacks specificity for cancer cells and is inherently toxic. However, it is important to recall that it was not so long ago that cancer was almost universally regarded with great pessimism as completely untreatable – irradiation for throat cancer, platinum derivatives for ovarian and testicular tumours, and combination chemotherapy for several of the cancers of childhood have tempered this gloomy view. The fact that there have been some remarkable successes is something of a triumph of modern medicine and deserves emphasis. But what we really need is an explanation.

Why are some disseminated cancers very responsive to treatment and others – unfortunately, the majority – very intractable? Why are the cancers of childhood more curable than those of adults? The answer lies in the genetics and biology of the disease, something which until recently was hidden from view.

As we have now seen, the cancer clone can, over time, generate very large numbers of cells, is often genetically unstable, defective in DNA repair, and may have lesions in the cell death pathway. And, most significantly, in the context of attempts at eradication, the clone is hyperdiverse and remarkably plastic in its adaptability. It is a highly predictable consequence of the clonal evolution of cancer that once graduation to metastasis has occurred, at least a few cells within the emergent clone will escape therapeutic assault and resurrect clonal dominance. How they do so is no longer a mystery; the tricks of the trade are, at least, now exposed.

Before we deal with cancer cell perfidy, we need to acknowledge one or two false assumptions that have underpinned our approaches to treatment. A common premise has been that cancer cells grow more quickly than normal. It isn't necessarily so. Unfortunately, the belief that it was provided the basis for mainstay systemic therapy with drugs and radiation that preferentially kill any rapidly dividing cells. It turns out that some cancer cells in fact divide very slowly – but persistently; dominance by stealth. This is true for prostate cancer, for example, as well as for a number of other cancers including some lymphomas and some breast cancers. Cancer cells can masquerade as superficially docile or even sleeping and so evade conventional therapy. This could be an accident of the developmental route taken by these mutant cells but more likely it is an adaptive Darwinian tactic endorsed by selection for slow but inevitable success. We just got it wrong here.

We have also been duped into believing, or at least hoping, that particular types of cancer classified into stages or grades of malignancies, could be treated clinically as if they were single or homogeneous entities. We can now see that a remarkably rich molecular diversity lies below the surface. Moreover, it is now clear from clinical studies in leukaemia in particular but also in breast cancer that the underlying molecular abnormalities singly or in combination can have a profound impact on the response to particular therapeutic cocktails. The outcome of 'molecularly blind' therapy is then variable, unpredictable, and largely disappointing.

Consider next the mode of action of non-surgical treatments. It turns out that most chemotherapeutic drugs and ionizing radiation used to treat cancer do not operate, as long assumed, as cellular assassins, killing with poisons or explosives. Rather they damage DNA, in response to which the cell activates its preprogrammed and suicidal cell death pathway. It's not murder but suicide, albeit prompted by assault. But as we have seen, this very same cell death process is already aborted by many mutations that contribute critically to the evolution of the disease in the first place: hence the likelihood of therapeutic failure. Of course all cancer cells will die if you give enough drugs or radiation at very high doses – but so too will the patient.

What then of the cancers that are curable by chemotherapy with or without assistance from radiation? I have argued that most of the few clear success stories in cancer therapy – childhood leukaemia in particular but also Wilm's kidney tumours in children, Hodgkin's disease, testicular teratoma, and chorio-carcinoma in young adults – are in fact exceptional examples of cancers which are suspected or known to originate from somewhat special stem cells and that have abbreviated evolutionary trajectories into diagnostic prominence. These particular cells, for sound developmental and physiological reasons, are mobile, actively proliferating, and less constrained by tissue architecture but very sensitive to apoptosis and exit via differentiation. They may therefore evolve to a disseminated state prompting symptoms, diagnosis, and instigation of treatment relatively early in their evolutionary history with only a few mutations (say two for the sake of argument) and without the help of genetic instability. They may even, in my view, escape as disseminating cancer clones without the benefit of mutations that corrupt cell proliferation control or apoptosis, contradicting what has become something of a paradigm in cancer biology. These particular cancers are then intrinsically sensitive to drugs and irradiation and clinical cure is possible – provided, that is, diagnosis is not too delayed. These cancers too, if given the opportunity, will travel through an increasingly selective landscape and will generate further mutant diversity and, eventually, intransigent species. It's all in the timing.

So, good news and serendipity for some types of cancers, although, to be fair, therapeutic success did not come quite as easily as I imply. This interpretation of the curable exceptions has an important corollary: a potential explanation of the mystery of why we have had such a tough time dealing with most of the major epithelial cancers of adults. The latter evolve over much longer periods in the context of a tissue architecture which imposes formidable constraints; getting through this bottleneck to expand and metastasize probably necessi-tates increased diversification and the co-option of mutant genes for survival which allows the very rare successful escapees not only to set up camp elsewhere but, as a side-effect or bonus, to resist therapy.

But a straightforward block to the natural death programme in most metastatic adult cancers is not the only problem for therapy. Cancer cells that are defective in detection and repair of DNA damage (the evolutionary accelerator) are more likely to be, and almost invariably are, more resistant to therapy that depends upon DNA damage as the route to cell death. Up to 50 per cent of advanced, metastatic cancers have deletions or mutations resulting in loss of normal function in the *p53* molecule (our key cellular detector of DNA damage and conductor of the cell death programme). The instigation of therapy may provide any silent *p53* mutants with just the selective opportunity they need to emerge as dominant subclones, following decimation of their competitors. This explains why the absence of normal *p53* function in a tumour is usually predictive of further intransigence and poor outcome. Therapy in this context may even make matters worse by inducing further mutations in cells that are impervious to damage and don't therefore activate the fail-safe death option. In marked contrast, the sensitive and curable cancers referred to above seldom have *p53* mutations, probably because they have not been subject to the kind of selective pressure that encourages the emergence of this kind of mutant.

Unnatural selection

And, as if that wasn't enough, there is 'classical' drug resistance, long considered by cancer pharmacologists to be their only or major therapeutic hurdle. Here we really run up against the power of Darwinian selection, though in this case it is in a sense not 'natural' but an artefact of therapeutic intervention – but a powerful selective force nonetheless. The more cells there are (say 10^{12} or a kilogram's worth) in a metastatic cancer, and the more genetic shuffling or diversification that has gone on, then the more likelihood there is that silent drug-resistant mutants will exist prior to therapy. Many cancer drugs are synthetic or semi-synthetic copies of natural substances or xenobiotics, derived from bacteria, fungi, and other plants – in other words, naturally occurring toxins. And naturally enough, animal cells, including our own, have long ago adopted the trick of co-opting molecules that can neutralize, enzymatically degrade, or detoxify these microbial or faunal offenders.

If a cancer drug is going to work, then it has to saturate or overwhelm these molecular defences inside the cell. Providing cancer cells are sufficiently numerous and genetically diverse, (which is the norm for those that have metastasized) then there is a statistical likelihood that one or more of these cells will have, by mutation, improved its antitoxin defence. Treatment now provides the opportunity and selective pressure for these otherwise irrelevant mutants to survive the decimation bottleneck that strangles their siblings and to emerge as the newly dominant subclone.

This Darwinian process is essentially the same as the rapid evolution of insecticide resistance in six-legged pests – even to the extent that the same mutant tricks for escape have selective currency (for example, an increased number of copies of a gene that codes for a detoxifying enzyme). This mechanism holds for emergent resistance to most individual chemotherapeutic drugs. It also applies to antioestrogenic or antiandrogenic treatment in breast and prostate cancer, and helps explain why these cancer cells may escape by becoming independent of sex hormones for their proliferation.

A long-standing gambit to try and avert the emergence of mutant-based resistance has been to cycle drugs, as with antibiotics, or to use combinations. What success there has been in therapy of more advanced cancers has usually been with combination chemotherapy. It would seem unlikely that a mutant cell or clone would survive the challenge of multiple, different drugs filtering into the final cell death pathway by different routes and at high doses. But then comes the evolutionary rub again. Almost all our drugs used in cancer therapy, once in the bloodstream, rely on long-established normal cell membrane chemical pumps to get into cells: efflux as well as influx. Our cells use evolutionarily conserved mechanisms involving protein pumps and pores to encourage exit of such substances. Drugs that may have quite different chemical structures are recognized and are channelled through the same exit. These evolutionarily ancient arrangements allow cells to conduct a controlled dialogue with their toxic microenvironments and, in this respect, cancer chemotherapeutic molecules are perceived as part of a noxious natural world by a catch-all efflux trick that isn't a lot more sophisticated than a sluice gate. Unfortunately, this now provides an opportunity for a mutant cell, in one step, to gain resistance to several different drugs. This it can do if a gene for the exit pump makes more copies of the pump protein; efflux is stepped up apace, the cell and its clonal descendants become multidrug-resistant.

In all these 'ways of escape', the hardy mutant cell gains further advantage by way of the wholesale clearance and ecological decimation going on around it. Space and rejuvenation resources are then available for opportunistic ex-ploitation – as in parallel environmental catastrophes (forest fires, floods, asteroid strikes, and the like).

Other natural mechanisms, besides gene mutation or amplification, may also play an important part in imparting resistance via drug discharge. The ex-pression of drug efflux pumps varies widely between different cells of the body. For example, the blood vascular cells within the central nervous system are very well endowed in this respect and this probably reflects their function as front liners in the blood–brain barrier that prevents toxic substances entering our most vital organ. The same applies to the physical barrier of Sertoli cells that protect the testis germ cells from toxic substances in blood. Cells in the kidney, adrenal cortex, pancreas, and blood stem cells are also well equipped with pump proteins; this may explain why cancers originating from these cell types often appear to be intrinsically drug-resistant early on (that is, not the odd mutant creeping through the net but wholesale failure of chemotherapy).

Can you take any more excuses? There is one other reason why combination drug and radiation therapies are frequently frustrated. It has to do with local delivery. For radiation to work in killing cells effectively, there has to be oxygen around. For drugs to be delivered in adequate dosage to all cancer cells requires local diffusion from nearby blood vessels. I've already told you that a feature of evolving cancers is that beyond a certain size they solicit new blood vessel formation to improve their vascularization and nutrient plus oxygen supplies. It's now possible to visualize the often dense and extensive network of new vessels that surround and penetrate growing tumours, including their second-ary, metastatic deposits. New methods including microbubble ultrasound and fractal image analysis reveal that all is not well or as we had assumed. Rather than providing a symmetric, fine network of vessels, the new arrivals grow in an apparently haphazard manner leaving areas of the cancer distanced from vessels. These isolates will tend to be anoxic with substantial cell death but paradoxically within such regions, there is likely to be both selective pressure for the emergence of further mutants and dilution of the therapeutic attack. It's just not fair is it?

Clearly, the Darwinian odds are really stacked up against therapeutic success as the cancer clone evolves and expands. Much more so than we realized before the mutant genes and ways of clonal escape were identified. It really is no surprise at all then, now we see more clearly the genetic and evolutionary game plan of cancer cells, that chemotherapy for metastatic disease most often fails as some mutant cells, insulated from insult, escape through the most stringent of bottlenecks. No malign intent; survival of the fittest – cells in this case.

There must be some important practical lessons to be deduced from this story. But what are they? Some oncologists believe that more intensive chemo-therapeutic cocktails are the answer. Or, as Paul Ehrlich advocated almost a century ago with respect to microbial infections – hit them 'hard and early'. In modern USA parlance, this is 'up-front, mega-dose' therapy. No place to hide for any cancer cell then, no matter what its evasive, mutant credentials. There is a distant promise of some very fancy adjuncts to this strategy involving blood stem cell transplantation. These include gene therapy to make the transplanted stem cells resistant to high-dose chemotherapy and the 'manufacture' of new blood stem cells from the patient's own tissue (for example, skin cell nuclei) using a variation of the 'Dolly' cloning method. But these technically im-pressive cell and molecular engineering approaches are not offering new therapies as such. They are essentially tricks to rescue the patient from the potentially lethal consequences of very intensive 'old-fashioned' chemotherapy by replacing the essential blood stem cells that are inevitably destroyed.

These are then desperate measures, even though there have been some successes with dose escalation and 'rescue' with bone marrow transplants for leukaemia, and they might just work for some other cancers. But the trauma and collateral damage incurred with these essentially crude attempts to blast away the malignant clone is likely to be considerable, with no compelling reason to believe such therapeutic adventures have a reasonable prospect for achieving their primary objective. Others whose company I seek believe that we've been travelling too long now down the wrong road, blindfolded, and that this is no longer sustainable as a pivotal strategy. Of course if I was a cancer patient in a clinic today, I would expect to be offered the treatment that provides the best overall benefit and prospects for survival, even if it was toxic and nasty. But along with other potential rather than actual cancer patients, I also expect the options to improve – perhaps radically. The now well-recognized alternative goal is to adopt a much more biological approach to therapy that seeks to exploit our understanding of cancer cell tactics. Or, better still, stop it before it really gets up and running.

CHAPTER 25

EPILOGUE: CANCER IN THE TWENTY-FIRST CENTURY

If the causes for this variation (in the incidence rate of cancers) could be
identified and controlled, we could reduce the age specific incidence of the
disease by some 80–90%. Half of this could be achieved by application of
existing knowledge.

(Sir Richard Doll, 1996)

The evolutionary and historical picture I have tried to paint might
encourage a fatalistic trait of resigned inevitability. I hope not, because
that's not how I and, I believe, most cancer researchers (admittedly
inveterate optimists) now see the problem. Cancer is in one sense an inevitability, at a certain level. The height of that level for different cancers is
however a social variable. Understanding how cancer clones operate tactically
is one half of the battle won. We can tackle the clone more cleverly or we can
confront the social ratchet that escalates risk; or we can try to do both. It surely
has to be both, but there are choices and priorities to be made. There still will
not be a 'magic bullet', however sophisticated, for cancer in general. Political
leaders and advisers should now recognize that the problem isn't equivalent to
the task of building the first atomic bomb and getting a man on the moon. The
intricacies of millions of years of evolutionary biology are involved, richly
embroidered and coupled in conflict with human diversity and behaviour.

Great expectations

So what can we do to exploit our new biological knowledge? Several enticing
possibilities exist and some have already progressed into early clinical trials.
There is much optimism that some of the new molecular strategies will prove
effective. Entrepreneurs and biotechnology companies can see dollar signs
flashing, and this may not be a bad thing provided the eventual product costs
can be borne.

But will the goods be delivered? Lewontin, Cairns, and other sceptics of the molecular biology enterprise in cancer therapy have cautioned against extravagant expectations. The hype coming both via the media and from vested interests in molecular therapy of cancer and gene therapy in general could easily engender a resigned or cynical pessimism. We've heard it all before? So much is at stake that premature or exaggerated claims to boost stock value, personal, or institutional prestige are inevitable. Good news is what we all want to hear but it is grotesque to pretend to cancer patients that the answer, and a simple one at that, is just around the corner. In some respects, the deception can be even worse now that it can be dressed up in a cloak of impressive but largely impenetrable genetics and molecular biology.

On the other hand, who cares if entrepreneurs lose some of their money? Investment is unquestionably fuelling the extraordinary technological advances that make some forms of molecular therapy at least possible, and amongst them there could be one or two eventual winners. Governments and medical charities cannot gamble on such a scale alone and only a few academic cancer research centres worldwide enjoy sufficient skills and investment to take on the challenge effectively. In the meantime, what is Joe Public supposed to make of it all? Sober appraisals of prospects and problems are as rare as hen's teeth. There are real prospects; and there are real problems. It's not the purpose of this book to provide an in-depth critique of this important issue but the synopsis that follows offers a flavour of the challenge ahead, distilled out with the Darwinian credentials of cancer clones in mind.

Molecular horoscopes?

For those cancer genes that are inherited, sensitive and specific screening methods will soon be in place for screening high-risk groups (for example, for familial breast, colon, or prostate cancer). Knowing you don't carry the gene in question is very important and will be more helpful when we have a complete inventory of the culprit mutant genes involved. But if you do, then there is now a much better chance that early detection, surgery, plus perhaps dietary advice and hormonal prophylaxis (in the case of breast cancer), will stop the rot. Individuals with genetically confirmed familial cancer may well wish to avoid passing on their potentially harmful mutant gene either by choosing not to have their own biological children or by using IVF and molecular screening for mutant-free embryos. Of course, as with the many other inherited genes with potentially lethal consequences later in life, there are other serious issues to consider, not least the logistics of appropriate screening itself, risk assessment and counselling, treatment options, and life insurance cover. It's a little worrying that some biotechnology companies are showing signs of wishing to get into the market-place with potentially lucrative genetic screening tests before the necessary adjuncts are in place.

For the majority of cases of adult cancer in which powerfully acting, inherited cancer genes are not involved, individuals at greater risk may still be identifiable, for example via genetic variations in genes concerned with carcinogen metabolism, hormonal signalling, or the immune response. But the modulation of risk attributable to genetics in this sense is likely to be modest or the compound effect of many genes; this poses considerable problems for screening tactics and the potential benefit may be small.

More realistically, the efficacy and reliability of early detection of cancer itself by regular and systematic screening is likely to be much improved by the identification of mutant genes that signal escalating malignancy and by the introduction of effective methods for detecting them in early lesions. Sensitive and comprehensive molecular screening technologies based on microarrays are under way that can be used to identify mutant fingerprints in extracts of very small biopsies. The reasonable expectation is that a full audit of the molecular abnormalities should provide a more reliable measure of the evolutionary status of cancer clones. It will never be foolproof, however, because of the unpredictable nature of the cancer cells' evolutionary trajectory. Nevertheless, early detection in these circumstances should improve clinical prognosis and the chances of eradication.

Covert dissemination of the cancer clone may lead to delay in systemic drug treatment and therefore the application of molecular diagnostics applied to local lymph nodes, blood, or accessible body fluids may improve our identification of patients who need systemic as well as localized treatment. The mortality burden of invasive cancers could be reduced by screening, as evidenced by the experience with cervical cancer, and much more could and probably will be achieved in this respect. The trick has to be to catch tumour cells before they graduate into fully-fledged cancerous migrants. The challenge is to make the screening smart rather than sloppy, accurate, and available and then to encourage take-up by appropriate groups of individuals at risk. The implications here for technological innovation, resource provision, and public education are, to say the least, considerable.

Screening for breast and prostate cancer is where this issue is perhaps most contentious. Carcinoma of the breast, in common with other adult cancers, is a chronic disease, albeit one that can emerge from its largely silent natural history to become acute in impact. It ought to be possible therefore to design surveillance and detection technologies that can tease out tell-tale signs of the problem long before the full house of mutations, liberating metastatic spread, is dealt. Mammography has saved some lives in this respect but the overall benefit is at best modest.[2] The screening method simply isn't smart enough.

This should improve with scanning methods that promise to provide more informative images of tumours.

Similar arguments apply to prostate screening. In the USA, where the approach is more gung-ho than in Europe, regular screening is identifying many men at risk, but the risk is not as yet accurately quantifiable and many who might not develop life-threatening malignancy are losing their prostate glands with some considerable consequences. Provision of services for the scrutiny of incipient cancers would benefit greatly if linked to some capture of molecular profiles of mutant genotypes and prognostic predictability that can guide and rationalize intervention.

There are other encouraging developments in this respect. I do not particularly relish having an endoscope pushed regularly into my rectum, but there is now good evidence that so-called magnified endoscopy can efficiently survey the rectum and colon for suspicious lesions that might merit further interrogation by biopsy or removal. Colonic polyps of more than one centimetre in size have a high probability of evolutionary progression to more fully-fledged cancer and there is now compelling evidence that their detection and removal, by colonoscopic polypectomy, can reduce cancer incidence by some 90 per cent. Whether such a 'service' will ever have widespread availability as part of health service provision is perhaps debatable.

Dumping on the clone with 'designer' drugs

But prediction, accurate early diagnosis, and removal of solid tumour lumps is unlikely to be enough; we will still urgently need more effective, less toxic treatment of metastatic disease. It is inevitable that some patients will continue to be diagnosed only after their cancer clone has disseminated. Much technical wizardry is likely to be required if we are to finesse fully-fledged cancer clones. Can we induce them to die? Cancer cells may have their cell death pathways blocked but these are silent and inaccessible, not extinct. There is therefore a possibility that the process can be resurrected by delivery of apoptotic signals that bypass the normal cellular signalling entry routes; or mutant proteins that inhibit the cell death route might themselves be inhibited.

Interesting though these possibilities are, they beg an obvious question: how will this lead us to drugs that are selective for cancer cells and non-toxic? In a sense this is a real acid test for a century of cancer research: will it be possible to target or manipulate cancer cells via their Achilles' heels – their mutant genes, or the abnormally regulated protein functions they encode? Test-tube and some animal experiments suggest that it may be, but this is where much technical virtuosity will be needed. Billions of pounds and dollars are now backing this horse in anticipation that it will herald in a new generation of non-toxic, designer drugs and a new era of molecular therapy for cancer.

Now I'm sorry to be such a spoilsport but there is a real problem here also, and one that cancer molecular biologists often ignore. It's the perennial problem of specificity for the cancer cell. Paul Ehrlich's salvasan was the first 'magic bullet' almost a century ago. Its success was hugely dependent upon the fact that syphilitic spirochaetes are very different beasts from our own cells and so a very high therapeutic ratio of bug kill to cell kill could be achieved. Mutant genes may be cancer cell specific, as may the proteins that they encode, but the signalling pathways that they critically deregulate are not. What's special about cancer cells is their confusion over time and place. Molecular targeting of a constitutively activated cell proliferation pathway, for example, via some highly specific peptide inhibitor of one step in the signal cascade (see Fig. 8.4, page 66), may have little more cancer specificity than an old-fashioned drug that targets dividing cells. The therapeutic agent may be exquisitely designed for *molecular* specificity but will lack the critical *cellular* selectivity required in cancer treatment. Directing molecular or customized therapy into this noisy area looks to me like a tall order. There is however still much we have to learn about the intricacies of signalling networks in cancer cells and there could be some very beneficial surprises in store. I would be happy to be proven wrong here and I have scientific colleagues who are confident I will be. We will just have to wait and see.

Ideally, one should target the mutant gene or its primary protein product itself, as only they provide the potential of real specificity. To do so will require some very fancy footwork, but there are encouraging signs. The most prom-ising potential target molecule in this respect is p53. This is the protein that is lost or has aberrant function in about 50 per cent of advanced cancers. Lack of normal p53 function is the most common biochemical distinction between malignant cancer cells and normal cells. It has excellent credentials therefore for a therapeutic target. Recent research indicates that it may be possible to modify a common virus (the common cold-causing adenovirus) to selectively kill only cells that lack a functional p53 protein. The initial trials with this novel agent, referred to as a 'smart bomb' (rather than 'magic bullet'), are en-couraging. Other research suggests that mutant forms of p53 protein can be restructured into normal conformations by small peptide molecules that bind to the distorted surface of the mutant. Therapeutic administration of such peptides might then be expected to render cancer cells more susceptible to genotoxic chemotherapy. I can conjure up one or two reasons why these novel strategies might hit the buffers also, but I won't. They are such smart ideas, they deserve optimistic appraisal. We will soon know.

There are plenty of other molecular kites being hoisted aloft with some alacrity in the cancer treatment field. These include attempts to activate the immune system to recognize mutant proteins in the cancer cell – a reprise, in a new guise, of the long-running saga of cancer vaccines. Another novel idea is to tag conventional cytotoxic drugs in a 'pro-drug' form in such a way that they can only be activated in the presence of, say, prostate-specific genes. It might be possible to exploit the unusually hypoxic environment of many developing tumours by using drugs activated by low oxygen conditions. And then there is the intriguing idea of thwarting the cancer clone's immortality by inhibiting its molecular salvation – telomerase enzyme.

So will any molecular 'smart bomb' ever really work – or will we have more dud scuds? It is a tall order on several accounts and I see no point in a show of bravado here. Some cancer cells will invariably hide in inaccessible sites: effective delivery of a novel drug, however magic or smart, will therefore be difficult. Moreover, the targets are in perpetual motion. Once the evolutionary pedal is on full throttle and cancer cells numerous and genetically unstable, then the chances of some mutant cells escaping the axe, albeit a molecularly 'intelligent' one, are very real.

A Darwinian bypass?

Ideally, we should seek a treatment modality that abolishes or restrains evolutionary opportunity for cancer cells without at the same time providing the selective pressure that encourages the emergence of resistant mutants within the clone. This is an extraordinarily difficult and almost irreconcilable conflict for any therapy aimed directly at cancer cells, especially once they have gained a foothold and are genetically diverse and poised for escape. But there is a possible way round this problem. Intervention to prevent or restrain the transition of tumours or premalignant growths to invasive cancers, or even the expansion of metastases, may well become possible as we learn more of the critical biological mechanisms involved – tissue barrier breakdown, cellular adhesion, and, in particular, new blood vessel formation or angiogenesis. Herein lies one possible intervention that might just have widespread application in cancer – the prevention of new blood vessel formation in adults, without which there would be no cancer clone evolution: squeezing the bottleneck and suffocating the tumour.

This approach has a very appealing biological rationale. The major problem in designing any therapeutic bullet for cancer cells, magic or otherwise, is that their genetic diversity provides them with a means of resistance and clonal escape when confronted with the intense selective pressure of therapy. Aiming the attack on the blood vessels is not subject to this severe, Darwinian limitation, as these cells are genetically stable subordinates of the cancer clone. The idea then is to tackle, or shackle, the landscape that the cancer cell must travel through rather than the clone itself.

Will this approach have adequate efficacy and selectivity? New blood vessels are physically accessible for targeting – which is a good starting point. But then wouldn't a full frontal inhibition of blood vessels incur some penalty points? We need the capacity to generate new capillaries primarily to form a normal embryo, foetus, and baby, but why do we need this capability as adults? Well, it is required in reproductive females for cyclical function of the ovary and for the formation of the placenta in pregnancy, and is important in wound healing and inflammation, but otherwise it is a thorough nuisance, not just for cancer but for diabetic retinitis, blindness, and arthritis. Inhibiting angiogenesis might therefore be beneficial without the penalty of major collateral damage characteristic of most cancer therapies.

Following on pioneering studies by Judah Folkman and his team in Boston, a plethora of natural substances have been identified that block the proliferation of new blood vessels including chemicals in shark's cartilage and green tea. Some of these could have therapeutic potential and at the time of writing, at least 10 products are in phase I or II clinical trials, and others are in development. Some very promising candidates identified (for example, endostatin) also appear to be remarkably efficacious in animal models of cancer. Tantalizingly, one of the most potent antiangiogenic chemicals turns out to be thalidomide. It would be an extraordinarily bizarre turn of events if this drug had some useful application.

There will be difficulties however. Compounds like thalidomide operate by interfering with particular chemical signals – one called TGFα, in particular – and these molecules are not only important for blood vessel formation but for other vital functions including the immune response. There is certainly a strong incentive here to find a compound specific for blood vessels and it might be possible. It's probably the best new therapeutic card we have to play.

These considerations temper optimism but they need not abolish it. Even by the time this book is published or you are reading this page, much more insight will already have been gained and the likelihood is, on balance, that some very real practical benefits will have occurred via the biological route in terms of early intervention, restraint of tumour expansion, or, in some cases, permanent or at least worthwhile shrinkage of metastatic cancer. Beyond all the hyperbole, there is some very clever cancer science about.

In the meantime, there may be simpler options. There is now persuasive though incomplete evidence that non-steroidal anti-inflammatory drugs can reduce the incidence of precursor lesions in the colon and lower the risk of colon cancer, perhaps by 50 per cent. The same drugs can similarly suppress the formation of aberrant intestinal clonal growths in rodents administered with cancer-promoting chemicals. So what are these remarkable drugs? Well, one is a derivative of a natural plant substance used for more than two thousand years as a painkiller. Hippocrates recommended its use to women in the form of an infusion of willow extract for relieving labour pains. It has been manufactured for one hundred years and it is cheap. It's aspirin. And not only does it protect your colon and get rid of your headache, it is clearly beneficial for those at risk of heart attack or strokes.

This extraordinary versatility stems from aspirin's capacity to interfere with prostaglandins that are part of the signalling network controlling cell division and death. The net impact of aspirin in the intestine cells will be – division down; death up. Now, if any new cancer drug was invented with these credentials, and was covered by patent protection, don't you think there would be a real hullabaloo about it? And wouldn't you bet it would be very expensive? Aspirin is not the magic bullet by any means, and it can have unwanted side-effects, but it beats most other candidates out of sight.

Restraining the ratchet

All the wizardry of molecular biology alone will not be sufficient to resolve the cancer problem. Common sense dictates that prevention would be better, and pragmatically, this may ultimately prove a very necessary and major component of society's effort to outflank cancer. It won't be easy either but the potential impact is huge. My guess is that when it comes to cancer control, history will repeat itself. That, as with the control of infectious diseases earlier in the twentieth century, the battle will be won in part only by sophisticated science and, in larger measure, by remedies allied to living conditions, social and economic strictures, and lifestyle. By the same token, it is generally recognized that the biggest contribution we could make to health on a worldwide scale would be clean water. And nobody is advocating a return to Stone Age lifestyle.

The counter-argument is that widespread and enjoyable habits, especially when gift-wrapped in commercial profit and tax revenue, are unlikely to change and, anyway, it would take too long. This is a dangerously defeatist view. There are those who resent the very idea that our behavioural patterns or lifestyle are major contributors to cancer risk. This, they assert, is blaming the victim. But there is no general sense in which individuals or society are to blame. This long-running bipartisan argument is facile and counter-productive. That some personal or lifestyle decisions are involved is indisputable but not in the trivial or ephemeral sense of choosing a hairstyle, make of car, or fashion accessory. We do not necessarily have complete control over the relevant behavioural traits and they are heavily biased by the social and

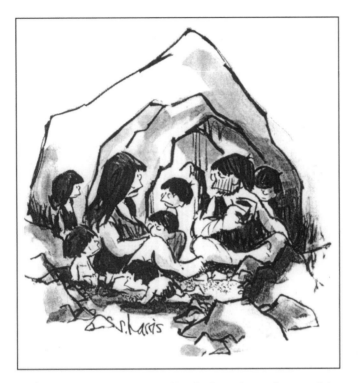

Figure 25.1 'How can we *prevent* pregnancy? We don't even know what *causes* it.'

economic systems within which we live and work. We may have a black-hatted villain in tobacco, but the forlorn search for a unitary cause of cancer, a simple linear cause and effect relationship, is dead in the water. In the great majority of cases we are dealing with a complex causal network of biological, historical, social, and economic factors from within which emerges the angst of cancer.

But then any fatalist can wear a convenient cloak of inertia. We all have to die somehow so why not embrace free enterprise, enjoy life to the full, and risk cancer? Why not indeed. The trouble is, cancer, on average, 'removes' 15 years of life; it can be a thoroughly nasty way to go and, on the whole, it would be rather nice to be able to make an informed choice. We should adopt more modest expectations of oncologists, surgeons, and physicians in terms of cure and place more emphasis on the role of our culturally determined risk factors. When we're told that 80 to 90 per cent of cancers are, in principle, avoidable, then we are all suitably impressed. When we get down to an appreciation of risks to individuals from particular aspects of social structures and so-called lifestyle, then the problems begin – acceptance of risk, weighing of risk, and practical measures to intervene to mention a few.

Smoking-related cancer provides the most straightforward case to advocate.

Forget all the details and caveats, here is the risk expressed in vulgar but real terms: for every 1000 young men adopting a life time habit of smoking, on average, one will be murdered, six will die in road traffic accidents, and 250 will die of tobacco-related deaths including lung cancer. If this was a prize-winning lottery, most of us would regard a 1 in 4 risk of hitting the jackpot as a near certainty – even if we had a long wait for the prize. Stopping smoking, it is calculated, would eventually reduce adult cancer levels by almost a third, as well as reducing other serious health hazards in its wake. Lung cancer in the West is already dropping in incidence, in males at least. In the meantime, female smokers are now experiencing sour fruits of emancipation and male mimicry; whilst Eastern Europe, Africa, and China are heading for monstrous epidemics due to the pervasive or, shall we say, malignant activities of cigarette manufacturers. It's madness to accept this and it's sheer hypocrisy for Western governments to claim recognition of the health risks whilst providing tax benefits to the tobacco industry, subsidy to tobacco farmers, and allowing advertising.

Others, who know to their cost the dangers of cigarette smoking, have continued to this day to endorse its commercialization and provide a veil of respectability – including the British Royal Family. Certain brands of cigarettes have for over a hundred years enjoyed the accolade of a royal warrant or appointment to serve His or Her Majesty. No doubt a service of sorts has been provided: the present Queen's father died of lung cancer and both his father and grandfather died of tobacco-induced lung diseases. Somewhat akin then to King Charles I's descendants sponsoring axe-smiths. Finally, at the turn of the century, the Queen's Warrant Officers have revoked their support for the Benson and Hedges brand. Against all logic, however, the Queen's mother (who is older still than the warrants) will continue to provide one to John Player brands.

There is a risk that those who pull no punches in their condemnation of the tobacco manufacturers and the smoking habit in general will be portrayed as being pious infringers of commercial freedom and personal choice. That there is certainly a psychology of smoking, driven pharmacologically by nicotine, is none the less real; for many smokers the habit is in charge. The habit is un-questionably pleasurable and acceptance of risk easily neutered. Comforting if illusory reassurance comes in the guise of either 'OK, but it won't get me though' or 'well even if it does, lung cancer is just another ticket in old age to the great blue beyond'. In the end, it comes down to information and informed choice for youngsters growing up in a world full of competing temptations and social and commercial pressures.

In a sense, the message now being promulgated in the West at least is simple: tobacco smoking quickly becomes pharmacologically addictive; it's a very dangerous drug; it's probably going to kill you one way or another; and, on average, you can expect to lose fifteen or so years of life and have a thoroughly miserable time towards the end. Oh, and by the way, it makes your breath smell and it will cost you a great deal. And fortunately, because cancer clone evolution moves in staccato style at a sluggish pace, even for those of us who are past our prime, stopping smoking relatively late in life can significantly reduce the odds that a dominant clone will breach the point of no return.

Other major cancers are also in principle preventable. Several, as we have already seen, involve viruses, including papilloma viruses with cervical cancer, hepatitis B and C with liver cancer, and Epstein Barr virus with nasopharyngeal carcinoma (NPC) and some lymphomas. These cancers are more prevalent in less developed countries including S.E. Asia, India and Africa. For these, vaccination must be, in principle at least, the preferred option, although encouraging condom use might well 'fix' cervical cancer (and a few other problems at the same time). Vaccine trials are, at the beginning of the 21st century, in progress with all these viral cancers and encouraging preliminary results are emerging – with liver cancer in Taiwan for example.

An important and encouraging precedent does exist for prophylactic vaccination against cancer – the effective elimination of a herpes virus-induced cancer in chickens, Marek's disease. Before the introduction of Marek's disease viral vaccines, the economic loss to the US poultry industry due to this cancer was estimated (in the 1960s) at around 200 million dollars per year. If we can do it for chickens, then why not for another species of flightless biped? For some viruses that have a few clear-cut routes of transmission, it may prove possible to reduce or eliminate the associated cancers by preventing exposure. For example, the human retrovirus HTLV-I causes an aggressive form of leukaemia in adults in Japan and the Caribbean. It is transmitted primarily via infected cells in human fluids (like HIV) – that is, in maternal milk, blood, and seminal fluid. It should be possible to put restraints on these routes, as the Japanese are in fact doing by screening all blood donations and by advising all pregnant mothers who are virus-positive not to breast-feed.

Some co-factors which may critically increase the risk of virus-induced cancers (such as fungal aflatoxin contamination of food in liver cancer) should also be amenable to control. All told, virus-associated cancers are ripe now for effective intervention. Along the same lines, combined antibiotic clearance of the common stomach bug *Helicobacter pylori* has been shown to produce regressions and possible cures of gastric lymphoma, and has potential for a favourable impact on gastritis, gastric ulcers, and possibly stomach cancer.

Clean water would take care of bladder cancers linked to bilharzia infection – in Egypt in particular. Cleaner water should reduce the risk of bladder cancer in areas where normal supplies might otherwise be contaminated with carcinogenic chemicals. In fact, simply drinking more water might, by virtue of simple dilution and flushing effect, reduce the impact of whatever bladder cancer promoting molecules lurk in urine.[3] Though if you have worries in the bladder department, it would be helpful not to smoke as well.

For skin cancers, including potentially malignant melanomas, the message is now getting across that prudent reductions in high-level, intermittent exposure to the sun, and especially to the extent of burning, will greatly reduce risk. Particularly so in the young. Additionally, we have the advantage that these would be cancers that are easily visible, detectable, and treatable before they become malignant. This is becoming critical as melanoma incidence rates have risen dramatically over the past 20 years; it is now the most common cancer of women in their 20s. Currently around 20 per cent of melanomas prove fatal and yet all are potentially curable by simple surgical excision. No one need die of skin cancer. Surveillance programmes and trials of prevention or intervention, aiming educational and other tactics at the young are in progress in the USA, Europe, Australia, and New Zealand. These are expected to produce dividends but it will be two or three decades before we know for sure what the overall impact of these measures will be. In the meantime, as the incidence of melanoma continues to rise for at least another decade, some prudence in sun exposure is called for. And it's simply not enough to smother yourself in barrier creams whilst continuing to invite the sun's invisible rays to cook you medium rare.[4]

The evidence linking breast cancer with modern reproductive patterns and with diets rich in calories but impoverished in antioxidants, coupled with exercise deficits, may be incomplete but we expect more from epidemiology than it can reasonably be expected to deliver in this context, particularly since other dietary factors may modify risk downwards. Overall the evidence is persuasive, even though it may be only part of the total picture for breast cancer aetiology. A return to primitive Eve's social and reproductive lifestyle is not an option; hormonal manipulation to reduce the proliferative stress to breast tissue may be. It ought to be possible to produce a prophylactic pill for all females, post-puberty, that mimics the protective effect of early pregnancy. This tactic has already been shown to work in rats given the hormone gonadotropin, or a high dose pulse of oestradiol plus progesterone.[5]

Tamoxifen as an antioestrogen is also a step in the right direction and its prophylactic use (for 5 yrs) has been reported to provide a 50 per cent reduction in breast cancer for women at risk in one large North American study. But it has a downside including, ironically, an increased risk of some other cancers. Newer and possibly more efficacious antioestrogens are, however, in the pipeline. A key issue will be what impact these compounds, including those like raloxifene which retain weak oestrogenic activity, have on osteoporosis and heart or circulatory disease.[6] The idea of controlling breast cancer via oestrogen manipulation has been on the table for decades and started with the less than ideal option of removal of ovaries. We clearly require more biological insight into the normal hormonal physiology of the breast, but this is on its way with a major emphasis on breast cancer research in the USA and Europe.

And then we are what we eat. Diet is undoubtedly a major player in the cancer stakes. The epidemiological evidence here is not, and can never be, unequivocal; the chemistry of plant foods has such a baroque-like complexity, especially when it collides with the labyrinthine metabolic pathways of our cells, that it is surely naïve to imagine that we can distil out a few 'protective' molecules or replace them with a pill. And even those plant molecules that do have protective credentials, for example the antioxidant flavonoids, not only come in literally hundreds of different flavours or varieties but are, paradoxically, genotoxic at very high doses. But the remedies are not necessarily complicated. The evidence that regular intake of fresh vegetables and fruit reduces cancer risk is very persuasive. A greater emphasis on diets enriched for these foods as well as fibre content, reduced in animal fat, and especially with diminished overall calorie content would make much sense and bring other health benefits, particularly if combined with a generally less sedentary, more calorie-burning lifestyle.

Snakes and ladders

None of these lifestyle manoeuvres can put a complete embargo on mutations in potentially cancerous clones. What they can achieve however, in this probabilistic process, is a very significant reduction in the odds that a full house of mutations will ever be accrued in the time available. If you don't smoke, moderate calorie intake as part of a balanced diet with regular fruit and vegetables, exercise regularly, and limit sunbathing, then lifetime cancer risk will ratchet back down. If there was a fancy pill that reduced cancer odds by, say, 75 per cent, you would take it wouldn't you?

These educational prescriptions for a healthy, cancer-free(er) society are already available, drawn up and disseminated by national cancer societies and other health concern groups. They are relatively simple and straightforward – almost to the point of blandness. Which is perhaps part of the problem. The average teenager in Glasgow or Detroit will consider them, if they are noticed at all, as 'naff' i.e. as dull, uncool, fuddy-duddy, unsexy. To a young man living in New York facing, statistically speaking, a more imminent threat from AIDS and homicide, cancer may seem a remote prospect. Youth culture being what it is suggests that some bribery, shock tactics and role models will certainly be necessary.

For a uniquely contemplative and supposedly sapient species of *Homo*, we can be remarkably dim and slow to take on board the likely consequences of our actions and, on the whole, inept at mentally weighing everyday risks. There are no doubt complex and interesting sociobiological reasons for this state of mind, some of which will be coloured with evolutionary or Darwinian logic. That we are a risk-taking breed is indisputable; and from this trait, great benefits and achievements accrue. Living in a risk-free world would be extremely dull and is neither achievable nor desirable. But the social game has changed.

In the rich, Westernized countries, most of us now enjoy the luxury of a ripe old age, access to health information, and financial resources. It makes sense now for us to pay more attention to unnecessary, habitual risks that can incur catastrophic if delayed payment – not much different in principle from having both the luxury and foresight to invest in pensions and insurance policies. And it's not just up to individuals. There are serious political decisions to be made on proper resourcing of health care provision. And cancer prevention should not be seen as an isolated agenda but a component of a generally healthier society; a quality of life issue.

We will need to get our act together. And soon. With ever increasing numbers of elderly people in Western societies, the potential cancer burden is escalating. Add to that a recent (2001) warning from the World Health Organization of the possible cancerous consequences of the increasingly adverse obesity/exercise quotients. Despite these demographic and lifestyle challenges I am optimistic about the likely impact of preventive measures, earlier diagnosis, and biologically smart intervention in the twenty-first century. My guess is that even if there were to be only modest improvements in the control of metastatic cancer, mortality from most major cancers in the West, including those of lung, breast, colon, and skin, is going to decline substantially. It will take time, since any benefit will not become fully transparent until several decades have elapsed (paralleling the normal evolutionary time frame of the disease itself). So by, say, 2025, I would expect the prognosis to be very favourable and by 2050 for the evidence to be indisputable. Cancer mortality will be drawn down in the future, just as the problem was exacerbated in the past, by social and socio-economic factors; and it will become apparent first in the better-educated and wealthier groups in society – notwithstanding that breast and prostate cancer control may still require some pharmacological assistance.

It is likely that the cancer burden will become more focused both in developed countries and, worldwide, on the less privileged – in other words, on those less able or less well-equipped to take charge of their lives and make the informed choices available to the rest of us. The social patterning of cancer will change, or rather continue to change. Several of the major cancers will decline in incidence or impact, as gastric carcinoma already has. But we should also expect that a few new ones will emerge or become more prominent.

Deaths from mesothelioma, linked to asbestos exposure of workers in engineering and building industries in the 1960s and 1970s, are still increasing and are not expected to peak until the year 2020. Uncontrolled use of asbestos remains common outside of Europe and the USA. Countries in South East Asia that have been the major importers of asbestos, principally from multinational companies in South Africa, will hit the epidemic trail of mesothelioma sometime during the twenty-first century. It's an ongoing scandal of some proportion.

We still have to traverse the period of our medical and social history when prostate cancer is very high on the agenda of concerns. If my very speculative theory for prostate cancer turns out to be right, then what are the odds that overindulgence in Viagra, by the over 50s, might increase prostate cancer? And as cigarette smoking declines amongst affluent societies, what about other recreational, 'lifestyle-enhancing' drugs? Marijuana may have some medical benefits but is not an entirely benevolent or innocuous substance. It contains benzo(a)pyrene and other very dodgy chemical carcinogens. Moreover, at least one report has now demonstrated that smokers of both marijuana and crack cocaine have an increased frequency of molecular aberrations in their bronchial epithelium that parallel those seen in cigarette smokers. The same issues may then arise for cancer risk – how much you smoke or inhale and for how many years. Other unlikely but not implausible scenarios can be conjured up. If atmospheric ozone depletion ever arrives with a vengeance in the Northern Hemisphere, then the risk of melanoma will escalate considerably.

Liver cancer (hepatocellular carcinoma) in the USA has almost doubled in incidence in the 1990s, compared with just 10 to 15 years earlier, and looks set to continue to increase for a while. The increase was most marked in relatively young men and is most plausibly ascribed to increased transmission of hepatitis B and C virus in the late 1960s and 70s via intravenous drug abuse coupled with needle re-use, transfusion of unscreened blood, and unsafe sex – a sad parallel with HIV. Rates of infection have recently declined and so, in a delayed reaction, will cancer rates.

And finally, there is the disturbing trend in the West of increasing rates of oesophageal cancer, especially in men. Epidemiologically, the causal link is with alcohol consumption, especially when used in conjunction with smoking. As long ago as 1926, it was reported that there was an excess of deaths from oesophageal cancers in the beer trade (innkeepers, bottlers, and cellarmen). But it probably isn't simply alcohol flushing down the oesophageal pipe that's important. As so often in the cancer business, there remains a conundrum to resolve.

The reality is that we have always had and we will always have cancer. Complete eradication of tumours and all life-threatening or metastatic cancers is implausible. But the patterns of incidence for different cancers will change and, overall, the mortality burden is very likely to decline in the West as history repeats itself, and as new medical dilemmas come to haunt an ageing, affluent society. And in this changing landscape nothing will weigh as heavily as patterns, world-wide, of cigarette smoking.

Finishing at the beginning

Ironically, when we come to cancers in children themselves, the picture is somewhat different. For the minority with a known inherited predisposition, parental screening or IVF and early embryo screening are possibilities, but this is irrelevant to the majority. Many paediatric cancers may arise as spontaneous DNA errors in our complex developmental processes and may therefore be unavoidable. Fortunately for several of these, though sadly not all, current treatment is effective – though nasty. Novel types of molecular therapy may have a major part to play here, for example, with brain tumours.

However, for the major cancer of childhood, acute leukaemia, there is new epidemiological evidence that it's top of the poll incidence may have much to do with modern lifestyle but not, as some would insist, from man-made radiation or pesticides. The thesis is that we have radically altered the way our infants become exposed to, and naturally protected against, common or endemic infections. Most infections that used to be acquired, at least in urbanized societies, by close social contact during infancy from older siblings, other infants, or mum herself are now delayed until playgroup or school times. These changes are linked to smaller, more insular family groups, improved hygiene, increased population mobility and mixing and have brought their own very substantial benefits in terms of reducing perinatal and infant infectious disease and mortality. But they may well represent an unexpected and paradoxical price to pay if delayed but common infection with some micro-organisms can occasionally produce severe proliferative stress in the bone marrow and leukaemia.

A similar paradoxical consequence of delayed exposure to common infections in the developed world may underlie a number of other 'modern' diseases including polio (the classic case), infectious mononucleosis (glandular fever), and possibly also Hodgkin's disease in young adults (a type of lymphoma), insulin-dependent diabetes, and multiple sclerosis. A similar scenario has been proposed for hay fever and other allergies. That such extraordinary and chaotic impacts might follow what at first sight seems a very beneficial change (that is, reduced infectious exposure relatively early in life) is, once again, possible because of a discordance between our inherent biology and our behaviour.

Our immune system has evolved to anticipate a challenge or assault from common infections around or shortly after birth, albeit in the context of protective maternal antibodies and protracted breast-feeding. There may also have been, during early periods of urbanization and increasing population density, selection and preferential survival of infants whose genetics best equipped their immune systems to respond rapidly and effectively to infectious onslaught. And, somewhat like a virgin brain, the immune system not only anticipates but needs an early confrontation with the microbial outside world as a learning experience to optimally model its pliable structure and prime it for later battles. It is not so well equipped to deal with later exposures in a naive state.

Current research is addressing the issue of whether childhood leukaemia does indeed involve an abnormal, delayed response to common infections. Its importance lies in the possibility that we might be able to prevent this cancer which has such a sad resonance, at least in developed societies. But why bother I hear you say; you've already told us it is curable and even why it is? The answer is that therapy for childhood leukaemia does not invariably work and when it does, the impact, trauma, and long-term consequences on the developing child can be very substantial. Children are extraordinarily resilient but we should not be seduced into thinking that things could not and should not be much better.

NOTES TO PART FOUR

1   Inequality of access to medical facilities is undeniably present in Western societies. There is evidence that individuals with cancer who are from lower socio-economic groups tend to present clinically with 'late' or with more advanced disease, reflecting some deficit in accessing primary health care and referral. Equally, hospitals vary in their success rates – more than health service providers and governments would care to admit or make public. This has to do with both provision and distribution of specialist resources and the accrual of experience in dealing with life-threatening illness and inherently dangerous treatments. In a recent (1999) USA study, investigators found that outcome for major coronary problems was significantly better in teaching hospitals with resident technical expertise than in non-teaching hospitals. Interestingly, a parallel study found that patients themselves felt that the non-teaching hospitals were superior with respect to emotional support. None of this comes as a surprise to those who have any familiarity with the structure and organization of health services in the USA and UK. A recent report (1998) from the USA Institute of Medicine surveys the issue and its implications for research spending and priorities of the unequal cancer burden on ethnic minorities and the socially deprived. The report is available on the Institute of Medicine website at http://www.nap.edu/reading room.

2   And contentious. See the editorial news section of the Journal of the National Cancer Institute (1999) **91**:750 for a recent discussion of this issue. And for a good general discussion of the logistical and technical aspects of preventive screening in cancer, see Cuzick J (1999) Screening for cancer: future potential, *Eur J Cancer*, **35**: 685–92.

3   For a discussion of the possible benefit of increased fluid intake in reducing risk of bladder cancer, see Jones PA and Ross RK (1999) Prevention of bladder cancer, *N Engl J Med*, **340**:1424–6.

4   Barrier creams may provide some protection but are not foolproof; they may also lead to a compensatory increase in 'risky' exposure. More effective screens or preventive topical applications may become available. Retinoid (vitamin A) derivatives appear to be very good candidates in the light of experimental evidence that they can prevent or enhance repair of UV light-

damaged skin (see commentary by Gilchrest B (1999) *Nature Med*, 5:376–7).

5. See Guzman RC, Yang J, Rajkumar L, Thordarson G, Chen X and Nandi S (1999) Hormonal prevention of breast cancer: mimicking the protective effect of pregnancy. *Proc Natl Acad Sci USA*, **96**:2520–5.

6. Jordan VC and Morrow M (1999) Taxomifen, raloxifene, and the prevention of breast cancer. *Endocrine Review* **20**:253–278.

FURTHER READING

Bailar JC and Gornik HL (1997) Cancer undefeated. *N Engl J Med*, **336**:1569–74.

Beardsley T (1994) A war not won. *Scientific American*, **January**:118–26.

Boehm T, Folkman J, Browder T, O'Reilly MS (1997) Antiangiogenic therapy of experimental cancer does not induce acquired drug resistance. *Nature*, **390**:404–7. With a commentary in the same issue by Kerbel RS (A cancer therapy resistant to resistance, pp. 335–6). And a cautionary note: Cohen J (1999) Behind the headlines of endostatin's ups and downs. *Science*, **283**:1250–1.

Borst P, ed. (1997) Seminars in cancer biology. *Multidrug Resistant Proteins*, **Vol. 8, No. 3.**

Cain JM and Howett MK (2000) Preventing cervical cancer? *Science*, **288**:1753–4.

D'Angio GJ (1975) Pediatric cancer in perspective: cure is not enough. *Cancer*, **35(suppl 3)**:866–70.

Doll R (1990) Are we winning the fight against cancer? An epidemiological assessment. *Eur J Cancer*, **26**:500–8.

Fidler IJ (1995) Modulation of the organ microenvironment for treatment of cancer metastasis. *J Natl Cancer Inst*, **87**:1588–92.

Gazit Y, Baish JW, Safabakhsh N, Leunig M, Baxter LT, Jain RK (1997) Fractal characteristics of tumor vascular architecture during tumor growth and regression. *Microcirculation*, **4**:395–402.

Giovannucci E, Egan KM, Hunter DJ, Stampfer MJ, Colditz GA, Willett WC, *et al.* (1995) Aspirin and the risk of colorectal cancer in women. *N Engl J Med*, **333**:609–14.

Greaves M (1997) Aetiology of acute leukaemia. *Lancet*, **349**:344–9.

Hahn WC, Stewart SA, Brooks MW, York SG, Eaton E, Kurachi A *et al.* (1999)

Inhibition of telomerase limits the growth of human cancer cells. *Nature Med*, 5:1164–70.

Hickman JA, Potten CS, Merritt AJ, Fisher TC (1994) Apoptosis and cancer chemotherapy. *Phil Trans R Soc Lond B*, 345:319–25.

Jain RK (1998) The next frontier of molecular medicine: delivery of therapeutics. *Nature Med*, 4:655–7.

Janssen WF (1979) Cancer quackery – the past in the present. *Sem Oncol*, 6:526–36.

Karp JE and Broder S (1995) Molecular foundations of cancer: new targets for intervention. *Nature Med*, 1:309–20.

Lowe SW (1997) Progress of the smart bomb cancer virus. *Nature Med*, 3:606–8.

Passalacqua R, Campione F, Caminiti C, Salvagni S, Barilli A, Bella M, *et al.* (1999) Patients' opinions, feelings, and attitudes after a campaign to promote the Di Bella therapy. *Lancet*, 353: 1310–14.

Peto J, Hodgson JT, Matthews FE, Jones JR (1995) Continuing increase in mesothelioma mortality in Britain. *Lancet*, 345:535–9.

Rosenberg, SA (1999) A new era for cancer immunotherapy based on the genes that encode cancer antigens. *Immunity*, 10:281–7.

Swisher SG, Roth JA, Nemunaitis J, Lawrence DD, Kemp BL, Carrasco CH, *et al.* (1999) Adenovirus-mediated *p53* gene transfer in advanced non-small-cell lung cancer. *J Natl Cancer Inst*, 91:763–71.

Twardowski P and Gradishar WJ (1997) Clinical trials of antiangiogenic agents. *Curr Opinion Oncol*, 9:584–9.

GENERAL FACTS, FIGURES, HELP, AND ADVICE

Sikorski R and Peters R (1997) Oncology ASAP. *J Am Med Assoc*, **277**:1431. This article shows where to find reliable cancer information on the internet.

For general information on cancer from the National Cancer Institute, visit http://www.nci.nih.gov or call the NCI Cancer Information Service in the USA(+1-800-422-6237).

For information on the genetics of cancer visit http://www.cancergenetics.org. This website was set up by Robert Lurie at the Comprehensive Cancer Center of Northwestern University, USA. It provides information for oncologists, other health care professionals, and patients.

BACUP is a cancer patient support organization with helplines. You can visit its interactive cancer website at http://www.cancerbacup.org.uk.

Can you avoid cancer? A guide to reducing your risks is an informative booklet produced by the Health Education Council, UK.

Avoiding cancer. The European code is a succinct but punchy leaflet produced by the Cancer Education Co-ordinating Group of the UK and Republic of Ireland as part of the 'Europe against Cancer' campaign.

Some national cancer societies provide information and advice on line and in booklet form on how to reduce risk of major cancers. They include the Cancer Research Campaign (http://www.crc.org.uk) and the American Cancer Society (http://www.cancer.org)

'Trends in cancer incidence and survival in the USA. Meeting "stat rites"' was published in the *J Natl Cancer Inst* and is based on the most current data derived from SEER Cancer Statistics Reviews 1973–1993; copy available at http://www.seer.ims.nci.nih.gov/Publications/CSR7393.

National cancer control programmes (1995) is a useful publication from the World Health Organization, Geneva.

'Guide to internet resources for cancer' is a website set up by UK cancer researcher Simon Cotterill. It provides links to many international sources of information on different cancers plus a link to a site enticingly called 'Quackwatch'. (www.ncl.ac.uk/child-health/guides/clinks1.htm)

A final word of caution: remember that anyone can put information on the internet and the quality of what is deposited is very variable.

GLOSSARY

Adenoma Benign form of tumour in epithelial tissue. May evolve to carcinoma.

Aetiology The cause of a specific disease (or the study of its risk factors).

Aflatoxin A toxic contaminant of some stored foods (e.g. nuts). Derived from fungus (*Aspergillus* group). May be co-factor in liver cancer in those living in humid countries.

Allele Alternative or variant form of gene.

Amino acid Subunit or building block of protein.

Angiogenesis The formation of new blood vessel capillaries.

Antibody Specialized blood protein made by the immune system.

Antigen Any substance recognized as 'foreign' by the immune system. Evokes cellular response and/or antibody production.

Apoptosis Process of suicidal cell death.

Benign Non-cancerous tumour that does not invade and destroy the tissue in which it originates or spread to distant sites in the body.

Benzo(a)pyrene Particular chemical constituent that occurs in tar products of burnt carboniferous substances (e.g. cigarettes). Damages DNA.

BRCA-1, 2 Breast (and other) cancer associated genes 1 and 2. Considerable increase in risk of cancer when inherited in mutant form.

Cambrian Geological period 545–495 million years ago. Time of significant expansion of all major types of multicellular animals.

Capillary Extremely narrow blood vessel.

Carcinogen Agent (chemical, ionizing radiation) that damages DNA and induces cancer.

Carcinoma Type of cancer, potentially malignant. Derived from epithelial cells.

Carcinoma *in situ* As above, but highly localized to single area of tissue.

Cell nucleus Central, membrane-bound zone of cell containing chromosomes.

Choriocarcinoma Cancer of the uterus. Derived from embryonic (placental) tissue.

Chromosome Linear structure of DNA and protein. 23 pairs of each in every human cell.

Clone Group of cells (or individuals) derived from a single ancestor. Term also applied, as a verb, to the synthetic production of multiple copies of a gene (or individual cells or organisms) by genetic and cellular engineering methods.

Cytochrome p450 Class of enzymes involved in oxidative metabolism (change) of carcinogenic molecules.

Deletion Loss of part or whole of gene or chromosome.

Differentiation Process of development in which unspecialized cells or tissues become specialized. The resulting cell may perform its function and die shortly thereafter (e.g. red blood cell) or cease dividing but function over many years (e.g. muscle or nerve cell).

DNA Deoxyribonucleic acid. The essential genetic material which controls heredity. Exists in two complementary strands wound together into a double helix. Packaged into individual chromosomes.

Encoding Basic function of genes; to carry coded instructions.

Enzyme A protein that, in small amounts, speeds up the rate of a biological reaction without itself being used up in the reaction.

Epithelium The tissue that covers the external surface of the body and lines most hollow structures.

Gene Basic unit of genetic code (DNA) that contains information for the formation of a protein or subunit thereof.

Genetic code The information carried by DNA that determines the sequence of amino acids in every protein. Thereby controls the nature of all proteins made by the cell.

Genome The total genetic (DNA) content of an individual or species.

Genotype Unique gene set for any individual.

Germ cells Specialized cells giving rise to sperm or ova.

HBV Hepatitis B virus. Common virus associated with liver cancer. Usually transmitted via blood.

Histopathology Standard diagnostic method for assessing type and grade of tumour. Microscopic examination of biopsy sections. May be augmented by staining tissue section with dyes or other reagents (antibodies or molecular probes).

HIV Human immunodeficiency virus.

HLA Histocompatibility locus antigens. Cell surface proteins that differ between individuals and initiate rejection reactions in transplants. Normal function is to facilitate recognition of foreign antigens (e.g. microbial) by the immune system.

Hominid Of human lineage (Homo genus or group of species including *H. sapiens, H. erectus, H. neanderthalensis*).

HPV Human papilloma virus. Large family of common viruses. Some types associated with cancer.

HTLV Human T lymphotrophic virus. Common variety, I, associated with a form of adult leukaemia in Japan and the Caribbean region.

Hyperplasia Reversible increase in cell proliferation in tissue. If persistent, can sometimes develop into tumorous growth.

Inflammation Natural tissue reaction to injury or infection. Involves infiltrating white blood cells and vascular (blood capillary) responses.

Ionizing Property of conferring charge (by electron transfer) on 'recipient' molecules e.g. by many, but not all, forms of radiation.

Leukaemia Group of cancers derived from white blood cells.

Lymphocyte Type of white blood cell (leucocyte) and key functional cell of the immune system. Two varieties, B and T, produce antibodies or destroy infected cells respectively.

Lymphoma Group of cancers derived from lymphoid tissue (e.g. lymph nodes).

Malignant Clinical term for life-threatening cancer. Usually applied to cancers that have become disseminated.

M.I.T. Massachusetts Institute of Technology.

Mastectomy Surgical removal of breast.

Melanoma Type of cancer derived from melanin pigment-producing skin cells. Can become very malignant if not detected and removed early enough.

Metastasis The spread of cancer cells from point of origin to other sites in the body.

Metazoan Collective name for all multicelled animals.

Monoclonal Derived from a single cell.

Mutation A change in the genetic material (DNA) of a cell, or the change this causes in a characteristic of the individual, which is not caused by normal genetic processes. Depending upon how subtle or otherwise the change is, the impact (on the encoded protein) will be neutral, deleterious (loss of one or more functions), or, very occasionally, beneficial (improvement in function).

Neolithic New Stone Age of human development (10 000 BC to 5000 BC).

Nucleotide A compound consisting of a nitrogen-containing base linked to a sugar and a phosphate group.

Nucleotide base Essential subunit of genetic code in all genes, consisting of adenine, thymine, cytosine, or guanine (A, T, C, or G).

Oestrogens Collective description for female steroid sex hormones (oestradiol is major type).

Oncogene Term applied to mutant gene that contributes directly and positively to cancerous conversion of cell.

Palaeolithic Old Stone Age of human development from 250 000 years ago to 10 000 BC.

PAP test Cervical smear sample analysed microscopically for abnormal, potentially cancerous cells. Named after its inventor, Dr G Papanicolaou.

Parasite Organism that exists by colonizing and damaging another.

Phenotype Unique, composite features of a cell or individual.

Pleistocene Geological period or epoch (1.75 million to 10 000 years ago).

Polymerase chain reaction (PCR) Ingenious, Nobel Prize winning technique for using nucleotides (oligonucleotides) and an enzyme (polymerase) to make millions of copies of the same DNA sequence. Can be used to detect very small numbers of copies of a gene (or gene fragment) and therefore of great value in diagnostic medicine and forensic science.

Polyp Tumour projecting from surface of tissue (epithelium or epidermis).

Protein Molecular end-product of our genes and the major functional and structural component of cells.

p53 Protein 53 (= 53 dalton in molecular weight). Important protein in protecting cells from stress or DNA damage. Commonly deleted or mutated in cancer.

p53 Gene encoding p53 protein (note: italicized for gene, roman for protein; similarly for all genes and their protein products).

Pyrolysis The chemical process of burning.

Radon Radioactive gas. Natural product of uranium decay in some rock formations.

RAS Gene commonly mutated in many forms of cancer. Encodes a protein involved in intracellular signalling and growth control.

Receptor Protein molecule that binds to partner molecule (or 'ligand') in a 'lock and key' fashion.

Sarcoma Group of cancers derived from 'supportive' tissues, e.g. connective tissue, muscle, or bone (osteosarcoma).

Senescence Ageing process in cells resulting in cessation of proliferative activity and dormancy or cell death.

Squamous Descriptive term for flat and scalelike epithelial cells or tumours derived thereof.

Stem cell Founder cell of specialized cells such as blood, epithelia, epidermis, and liver. Sustains production of such cells or tissues. Major target for many types of cancer.

Suppressor gene Gene that inhibits cancerous transformation in cell. Normally directly restrains proliferative activity or induces alternative activities (e.g. senescence, differentiation, or death). Loss of proper function of such a gene (via deletion or mutation) contributes to collective mutation in cancer cells.

Testosterone The main male steroid sex hormone or androgen. Produced principally by the testes.

Toxic/toxicity Damage to tissue.

Transgenic Animal, plant, or cell bearing an artificially transferred gene (transgene).

Translocation Movement or relocation of genetic material from one chromosome to another. Common mutational mechanism observed in blood cell cancers and sarcomas.

Uterine Derived from the womb or uterus.

INDEX

Terms defined in the Glossary are printed in **bold type**